# The COOL GIRL'S Guide to the FODMAP DIET

THE COOL GIRL'S GUIDE TO THE FODMAP DIET
EVERYTHING YOU NEED TO KNOW ABOUT (AND BEAT!) DIGESTIVE ISSUES FOR LIFE

Bentson Health Publishing
2597 Schoenersville Road
Suite 308
Bethlehem, PA 18017

The content provided in the book is not intended to prevent, diagnose or treat any disease; it is for informational purposes only. This publication is not a substitute for professional or medical advice, diagnosis or treatment. You are strongly urged to seek advice of a physician for any medical questions or concerns.

Ordering Information:

Special discounts are available on quantity purchases by corporations, associations, educational institutions and others. For details, contact the publisher at the address above. Orders by U.S. trade bookstores and wholesalers, please contact Bentson Health Publishing by Telephone: (610) 868-6800 or Fax: (610) 868-6806.

Printed in the United States of America

First Printing 2018

Cover and Book Design by Bentson Health Publishing
Editing by Dana Baardsen
Food Styling by Pauline Bonnet de Kerdrel
Food Photography by Pauline Bonnet de Kerdrel
Special Thanks to Emily Pellegrino

ISBN: Print 978-1-7324502-0-2 | eBook 978-1-7324502-1-9

# The
# COOL GIRL'S
## Guide to the
# FODMAP DIET

### EVERYTHING YOU NEED TO GET SAVVY ABOUT
### (AND BEAT!) DIGESTIVE ISSUES — FOR LIFE

## DR. KRISTEN BENTSON

FOOD STYLING AND PHOTOGRAPHY
BY PAULINE BONNET DE KERDREL

EDITED BY DANA BAARDSEN

**BENTSON HEALTH**
publishing

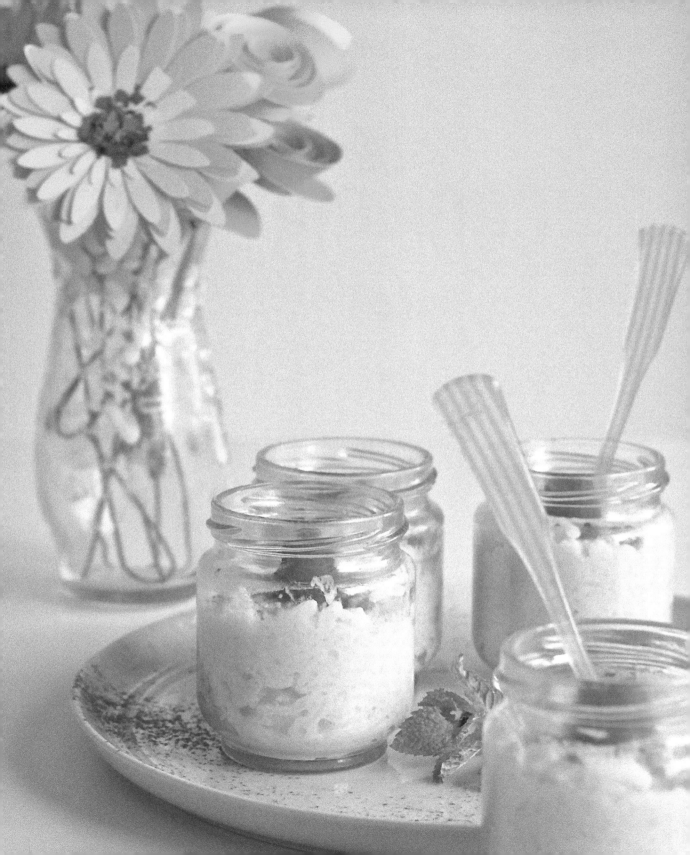

for my dad

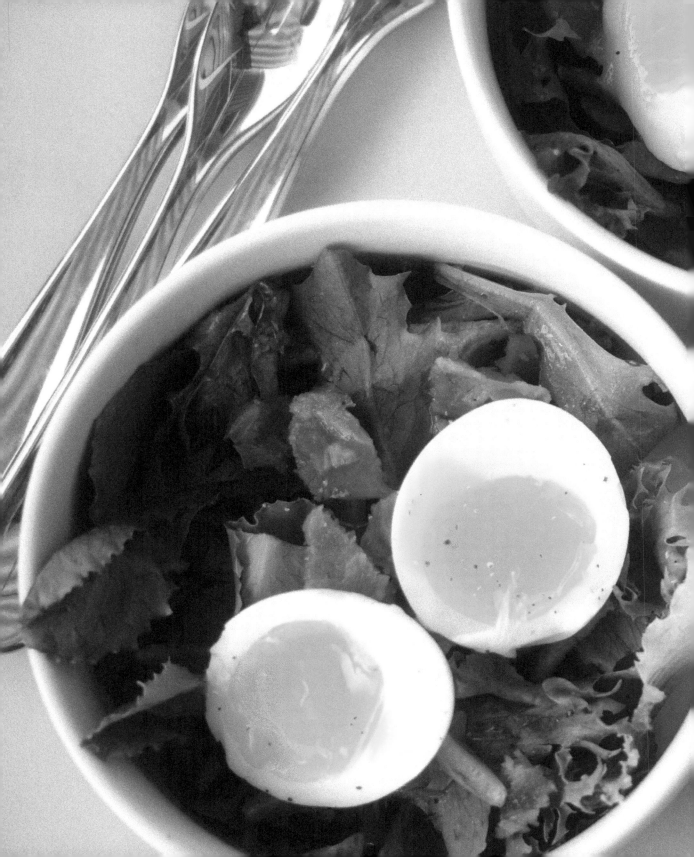

# CONTENTS

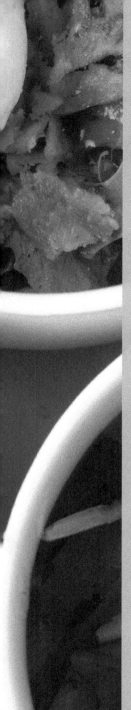

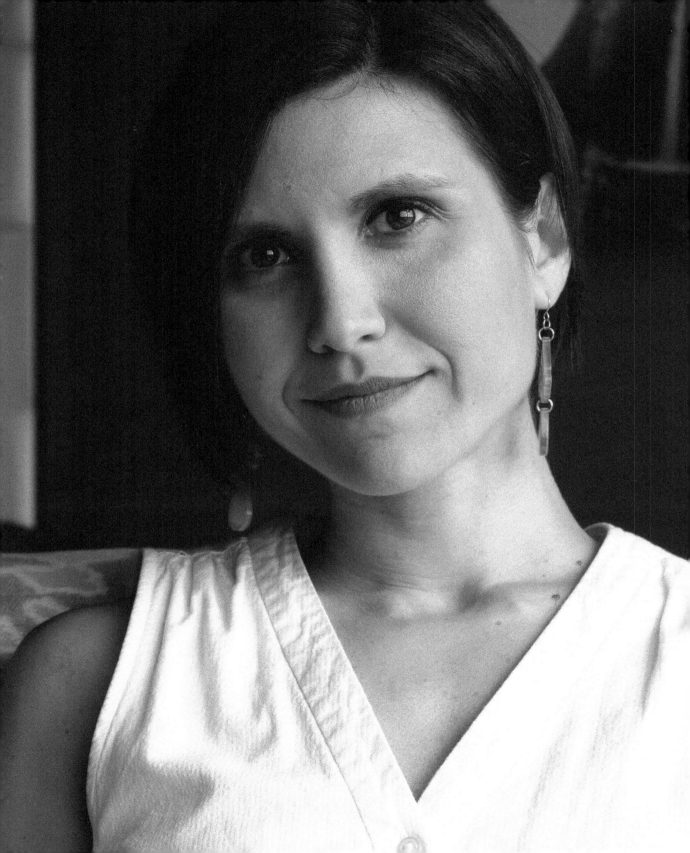

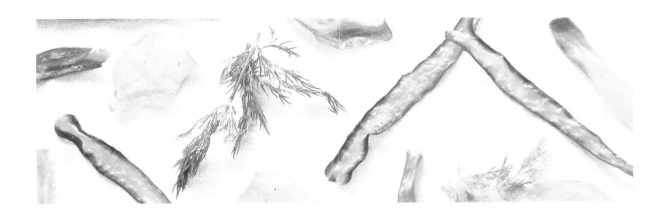

# INTRODUCTION

Ever been told or think you might have an irritable bowel? It's no joke! You'll find yourself squeezing into pants that constantly need to be unbuttoned, living in oversized shirts, rushing to the bathroom, and sometimes, even curled up in a ball on the floor in pain. The most frustrating part of it all? Chances are you don't even really know *why*.

If this sounds like you (or someone you love!), I've got some potentially life-changing information to share with you. Australian researchers have discovered the answers that "irritable bowel" sufferers have been looking for — it's called the low FODMAP diet, and it's like finally having a flashlight in a really dark room. Suddenly, you'll be able to expose all of those foods that cause your symptoms and illuminate the way to a lifestyle of purposeful eating that will leave you feeling fabulous.

By changing the way you approach food, you can change your life. I can show you how to recognize your triggers and eat mindfully so you can eliminate cramps, decrease pain, minimize bloating, and regain total control of your body. Let's get your digestive system working for you again!

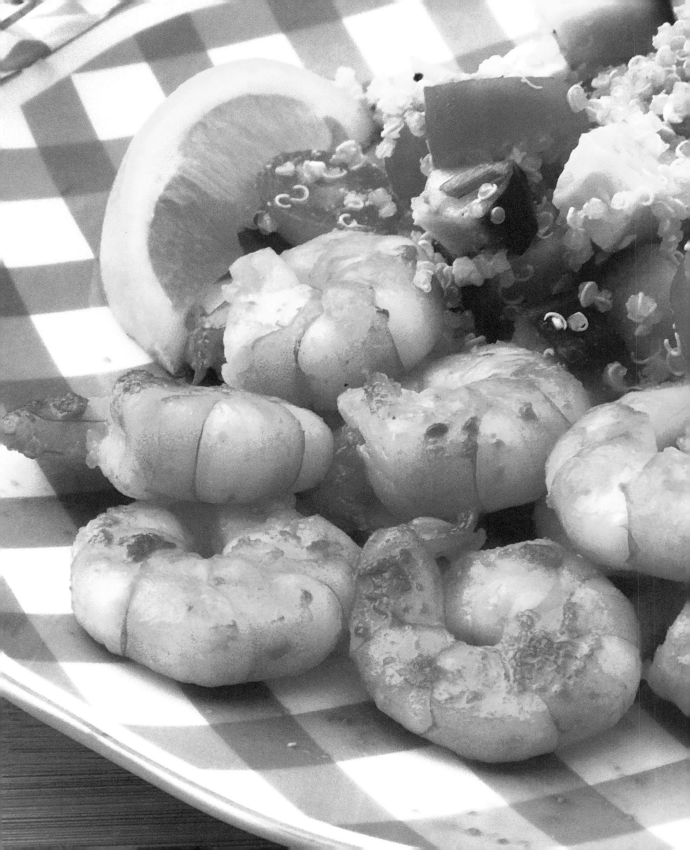

# FEEL FODMAP FABULOUS

*If digestive issues are (unfortunately) your thing and you're ready to make healthy happen, the low FODMAP approach to eating might be exactly what your body needs.*

It's good to feel cool, right? You know what I'm talking about — those glory moments when you're feeling confident, fun, and fabulous. But when you've got gut issues, feeling cool can be tough. Plus, being bloated and gassy almost always comes hand-in-hand with a crabby mood (*so not cool!*). If your bowel is irritable, chances are you'll be irritable too. And I get it — in those moments, it's easy to feel like antisocial weak-sauce.

The good news? When your digestive system is doing its thing, and doing it the right way, you'll feel like your coolest self. Trust me, it will feel incredible when IBS-related issues go away for life (*Poof! Be gone!*), and you're left with the strongest and most confident version of you.

I want you to:

- ☐ Say "yes" to that party or first-date without fearing your stomach might explode
- ☐ Feel confident walking into an important afternoon appointment without gas pain
- ☐ Go out to eat without scoping out the nearest bathroom before you even sit down
- ☐ Focus on your family event without focusing on your bloated belly
- ☐ Wear pants that you won't need to unbutton as the day goes on

I'm guessing you get what I'm talking about, and if you get it, I want to help you *get over* it. I want you to feel cool all the time. Well, at least any time you want to feel cool, and I think food is the answer.

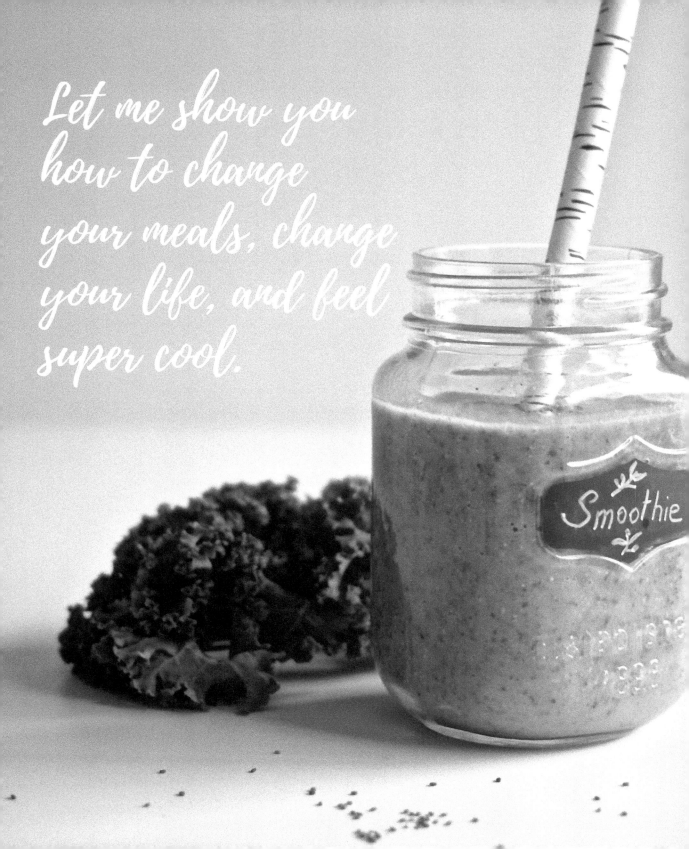

Let me show you how to change your meals, change your life, and feel super cool.

## SYMPTOMS OF IBS

Abdominal Pain

Cramping

Bloating

Diarrhea

Gas

Constipation

Indigestion

Nausea

## INDIRECT SYMPTOMS OF IBS

Anxiety

Depression

Loss of Appetite

Sleep Disturbance

Fatigue

Painful Periods

Pelvic Pain

Sexual Dysfunction

## BEYOND IBS

Not only is the Low FODMAP diet effective for managing and eliminating the symptoms of IBS, research is constantly evolving and this style of eating can also positively impact an array of other conditions. The low FODMAP diet can bring relief from inflammatory bowel conditions like Crohn's disease or ulcerative colitis. Studies also connect the low FODMAP diet with a decrease in fibromyalgia symptoms, and colicky babies might be soothed when their breastfeeding mom follows the diet.

So the need for eating a low FODMAP diet can be more than just a need to manage IBS.

Remember this: Food is never neutral, and it can never just be Switzerland! What you eat will either fight for you or fight against you. Everybody's body is different and responds differently to different foods. And while there are a bunch of foods that are terrible for you no matter who you are (*Hello added sugar, artificial ingredients, and GMOs!*), you've got to realize foods viewed as healthy can be bad for certain people at certain times. Just because a food is considered healthy, doesn't mean it's right for your body. That brings us to FODMAPs. Let me show you how to change your meals, change your life, and feel super cool.

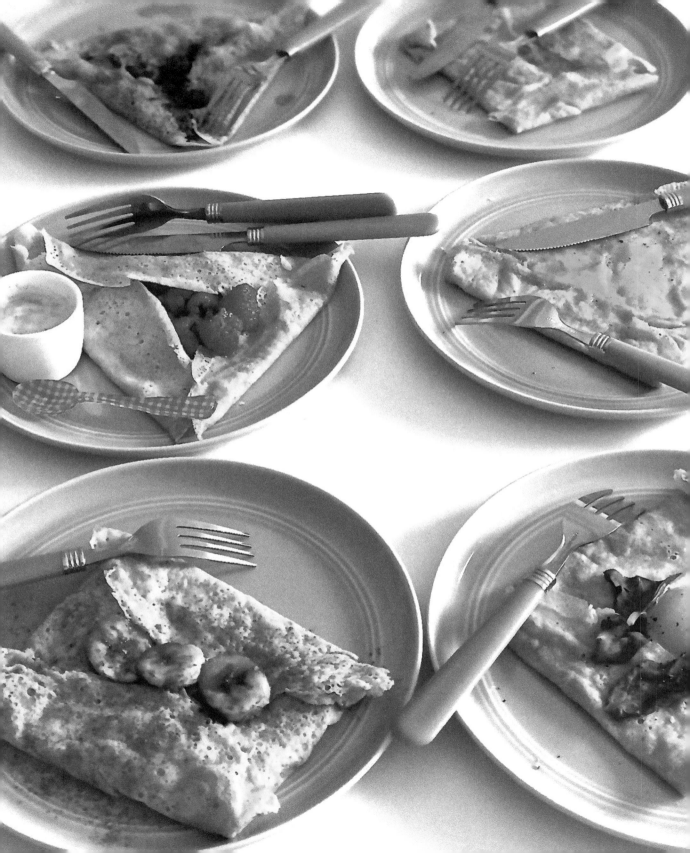

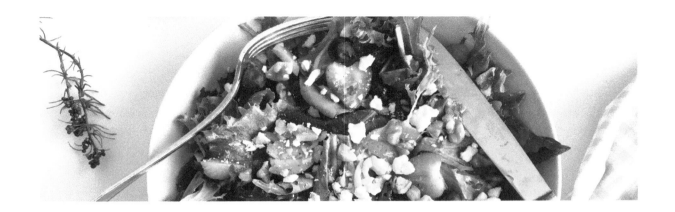

# TRYING TO FIGURE OUT FODMAPS? HERE'S HOW TO GET STARTED

For the longest time, experts in the field of gastroenterology have insisted that diet has little-to-no impact on soul-sucking symptoms like bloating, gas, diarrhea, abdominal pain, reflux, and irritable bowel syndrome. My opinion? I totally disagree! Food matters.

While in my 10 years of practice I have generally been able to help a lot of people reduce their symptoms, I'll admit there were times early on when I was stumped. For some of my patients, seemingly safe foods (according to the research of that time) would trigger abdominal episodes. Honestly, this was confusing and frustrating to me on a clinical level until I came across research out of Australia detailing the positive effects that a low FODMAP diet has on the most common GI (gastrointestinal) symptoms.

The big idea is that some of us (like one in seven people!) have a difficult time digesting certain carbohydrates or dietary sugars called FODMAPs, and most are women. Foods that are full of FODMAPs aren't absorbed as well and are easily fermented in the gut by the bacteria living there. The lack of absorption, and the fermentation that follows, creates a hot mess of issues in a susceptible individual's GI tract. Bottom line? If you're one of the sensitive ones, FODMAPs can leave you feeling miserable.

FODMAP stands for: Fermentable Oligosaccharides, Disaccharides, Monosaccharides, and Polyols. Basically, Australian researchers started testing foods to determine whether they are high, medium, or low FODMAP. And for anyone suffering from digestive issues, the results of their research is nothing short of life-changing.

*Eating high FODMAP foods can make an "irritable bowel" sufferer feel highly awful. Lowering FODMAP intake decreases the discomfort.* For a lot of people, it really is that simple. Are you starting to see why I'm so excited about showing you the ropes?

Eating high FODMAP foods (or even low to medium FODMAP foods in high quantities) can make an "irritable bowel" sufferer feel like their gut is — *ick!* — rotting. Why? Think back to your eighth grade chemistry class when you were learning about the byproduct of fermentation. Remember? It's gas. Excessive gas in your GI tract leads to bloating and distention (abdominal expansion beyond what's considered normal), which then activates pain receptors. *Ouch!* Gas can also slow down the GI system which can lead to constipation.

I've got one more pop quiz for you! Do you recall the principles of osmosis? It's when water travels from an area where there aren't a lot of particles to an area where there are lots of them. Well, when your body has all of those unabsorbed and undigested particles, water comes rushing into your intestines. Enter: Diarrhea.

The good news, your gut is spared the irritation when the foods you take in are low in FODMAPs. It makes sense, right?

Here's another cool thing: Researchers are finding the low FODMAP diet can actually increase the density of certain kinds of important cells, called enteroendocrine cells, that are found in the first part of your small intestine. People with IBS tend to have a lower density of these powerful cells, and more of these cells can mean less diarrhea and pain. That's just another reason to go low FODMAP!

As you get started, the goal is to focus on portioning and lower your overall FODMAP load. Think of a pot on the stove about to boil over. Add even just a pinch of something to that pot and the next thing you know, it's boiling over! The same goes for your "boiling" GI system. The first step is to bring your FODMAP "pot" down to a simmer. We'll do this together in the elimination phase of the diet. Once simmering, you'll work on systematically challenging higher FODMAP groups to determine which ones cause you to "boil." I call this the challenge phase — don't worry, I'll walk you through it. After you've challenged each group and determined which foods work for you and which ones don't, you'll reintroduce combinations of foods in the reintroduction phase. From there, you'll continue with an individualized and modified version of the low FODMAP diet that will work for you, for life!

In addition to helping others through my practice, my connection to FODMAP research is deeply personal. I've struggled with GI issues my whole life and have always been on the hunt for answers, not only for the patients I work with, but also for myself. So, I've put the low FODMAP diet to the test, and let me tell you, the results are incredible. It's official: You can use real, whole foods as medicine. You can heal your gut.

So, here's how it happened: I've always had digestive issues. In fact, I can't remember a time in my life when eating was easy and my abdomen *didn't* ache. Even from the time I was a kid, I recall running to the bathroom before even leaving a restaurant and staying in the bathroom for an awkwardly long time after everyone had left the table. After enduring several GI tests, I was told I had irritable bowel syndrome (IBS). The specialist simply said, "Eat more fiber and stress less." I was eight years old! I didn't have stress — I had a digestive problem.

Looking back, I realize most doctors at that time didn't even recognize the connection between what you eat and how you feel. I was stuck without help or relief, so I learned to live with it. I often found myself lying on the floor of the bathroom in pain and bummed to be missing out on yet another social event. Then, it all finally came to a head in college when my body started falling apart. My symptoms had become severe and incapacitating. I chose to seek out medical attention, again.

Finally, after 18 years, a doctor diagnosed me with celiac disease and a milk protein intolerance. I finally found some relief! I stopped eating gluten and dairy and I started getting better. While today celiac is easily identified, at the time I was diagnosed, it wasn't. Oh, and there definitely weren't any packages of gluten-free food or gluten-free restaurants for people like me. Being gluten-free wasn't popular, but I could have cared less that it wasn't socially understood. At that point, I only cared that I felt better when I ate better.

For a long time, my gluten-free and dairy-free life was awesome. The best part? After journeying through my health issues, I became excited and passionate about natural and alternative medicine. I convinced Scott, my husband (who was my fiancé at the time), to change his career path and come with me to chiropractic school. We committed the next four years of our lives to what felt like nothing but studying the human body and the art and science of chiropractic. After graduating, I decided to pursue a bit more schooling and finished up a masters degree in nutrition. Scott and I felt educated and ready to rock it out, so we opened up a practice together and dedicated ourselves to helping others.

Then came the babies — I had two! All was good until after the birth of the second one. I was dedicated to nursing my new little people, but along with breastfeeding came several (like many, many) rounds of mastitis, a wicked breast infection. With each infection, I needed antibiotics.

Now, here's where it gets interesting: In the months after having my second son, my digestive symptoms came back with a vengeance. I was sticking to my gluten-free and dairy-free lifestyle perfectly, but I was experiencing issues worse than ever before. Every day (by the time the afternoon rolled around), my stomach would become bloated, distended, and painful to the point where I could barely leave the house. The gas, pain, and digestive distress was beyond what I could take, especially while trying to run my practice and take care of two kids.

I couldn't believe it. *I was the food and natural health expert who couldn't figure how to get her bowel to stop being irritable.* I looked like I was still pregnant from the bloating and felt even worse. I tried everything. The only thing that helped was when I didn't eat, at all. I tried popular probiotics, which only exacerbated the problem. Little did I know at the time, probiotics often contain inulin, FOS, and other ingredients which are high FODMAP and often trigger symptoms! I tried a high-fiber diet, which made me feel worse. I tried an elimination diet, which worked until I ate an offending food — the random and frustrating part was that the same food that didn't bother me one day, rendered me incapacitated the next. I was at a breaking point.

At my lowest, my mom offered to take the kids for a few days. Scott and I were able to get away to one of our favorite cities, Washington D.C., and I finally had the time I needed to think straight. On our three-hour drive down to the capital, I ran PubMed (a website that indexes medical studies) searches and started diving into research trying to figure out what was wrong with me and how I could fix it. Then, I came across this interesting research on something called FODMAPs.

I sat in the passenger's seat reading (for the first time) about how high FODMAP foods can make an "irritable bowel" sufferer feel like their gut is rotting and how the gut is spared the irritation when the foods consumed are low in FODMAPs. It made sense.

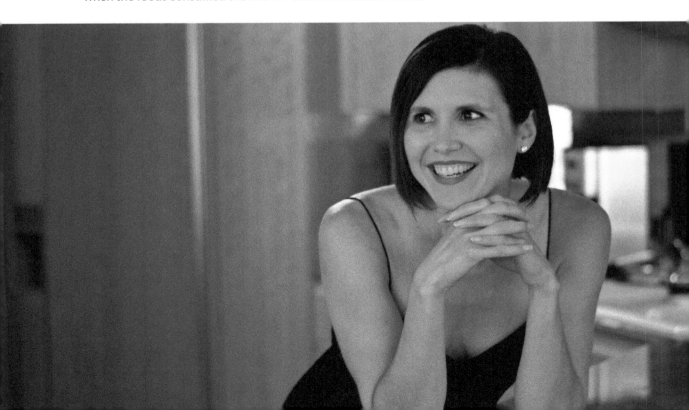

Guess where we ended up next? Whole Foods Market, the spot where my husband and I often grab a bite to eat. I loaded up my paper container with foods I was used to thinking were okay, like lettuce, chicken, cucumber, carrots, peppers, tomato, and sprouted chickpeas. Well, I didn't even make it to the bottom of my bowl before my belly started swelling. I was doubled over and thinking to myself, "Like, really?!" I wanted a fun night out with Scott and now the night was over.

Super frustrated, I thought back to that Australian research I'd seen while on our drive. I started Googling each of the foods I had picked up from the food bar to see their FODMAP status. Lettuce, chicken, cucumber, carrots, peppers, and tomato were all considered low FODMAP. Then, I checked on the sprouted chickpeas. Sprouted chickpeas are high FODMAP. This was my "aha" moment. I had finally made a specific connection between a food and my symptoms that made sense. I knew it was time to get serious about the FODMAP diet and turn myself into the guinea pig!

The next night, we hit up the same Whole Foods. I got the exact same meal, minus the sprouted chickpeas. And guess what? No pain! Like, zero pain, zero bloating, zero stress. To say I was thrilled is an understatement. Scott and I left feeling like we had figured it out.

*I want you to experience that same moment of pain-free elation.* I get it, it's often a journey and a commitment. I thought years ago I had it all figured out, only to have something new pop up out of the blue. Things happen, the body changes, and then you've got to change. But, I believe that everything in the body happens for a reason. If you can figure out the cause, you can effect the change.

*I am hoping you're able to do a little more digging to make healthy happen.* I'd love to say you can become healthy and pain-free by eating one specific food or by just avoiding another. But hear me out, there's no one thing that's going to help you to get healthy. Getting and staying healthy is a whole thing, and you're going to have to search in more than one place to uncover the answers you're looking for. The good news? Answers are out there — you've just gotta find them, and I'm here to help you!

And don't worry! I'll be with you every step of the way. I'll walk you through the elimination phase, the challenge phase, and the reintroduction phase of the diet so you can approach it with confidence. Plus, I'm going to teach you how to whip up some delicious low FODMAP recipes at home. You CAN do this.

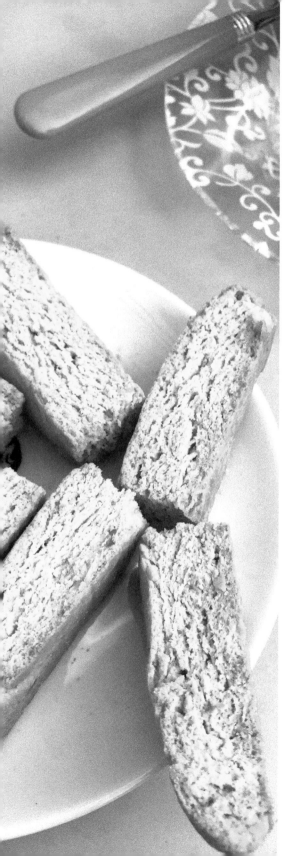

# WHAT IF YOU DID?

So what if you did go low FODMAP? What if you changed your meals and it changed your life? You've got nothing to lose but pain, bad bathroom experiences, and an unpredictable digestive system. But as much as it makes sense to simply try it, I understand that jumping in (and sticking with it) might feel daunting and a little scary.

I *hear* your fear. I know that changing your lifestyle and your approach to food is hard and that there are a lot of reasons why you might not even want to try it. I know there are foods that you feel connected to (that you love), and you just don't want to give them up. And, I know that your family and friends probably don't really get it.

I can totally relate, but I want to challenge your thinking. Right now, I am challenging you to replace thoughts of doubt with thoughts of determination.

Think about this: There are two purposes of food. The first purpose is to serve as a mechanism of coping with stress and the second is to protect you from boredom. Wait…I'm totally just kidding!

The first purpose is to give your body nutrients like vitamins, minerals, antioxidants, and phytochemicals. The second purpose is to give your body energy. When you set the intention to eat mindfully *and with purpose*, you'll start eating the nutrient-dense foods that are right for your body's unique physiology — you'll start to look, live, and feel your best. For you, this might mean eating a low FODMAP diet.

Social, emotional, and habitual eating aren't the answers to a healthy and well-functioning body. *You've got to stop living to eat and start eating to live.* When you do, food will become your greatest asset in the fight against dis-ease.

Henry Ford said it best: "Whether you think you can or that you can't, you're probably right." So, if you think you *can* find relief and feel like you *can* do this, you'll probably be right. Don't underestimate your mind-body connection.

I started telling myself this whole low FODMAP diet thing isn't really that hard. I convinced myself that I love the foods that I *can* eat. I told myself that I wouldn't be fazed by the, "You can't eat what?!" comments from unwitting food bystanders. I persuaded myself that this is doable and worth it — and rather than dreading the approach and the diet, I decided to love it and be grateful for it. I did it, and it changed my life. What if you did, too?

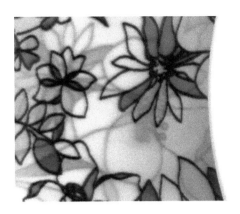
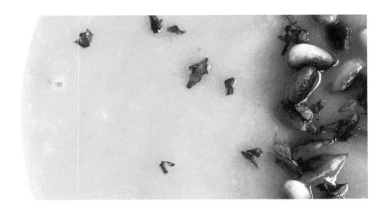

# ELIMINATION PHASE: FIND FABULOUS RELIEF

Sometimes, diets just feel so complicated. For this diet, there's definitely a learning curve, but I'm going to encourage you to keep it simple — eat foods that are low FODMAP and eliminate foods that are high FODMAP. Eat this way for four to eight weeks or until your symptoms are under control. Eliminating foods that are high FODMAP can totally reset your GI tract and promote healing. How cool is that?!

I believe it's so important to focus on what you can eat, rather than what you can't. While foods like asparagus, black beans, pistachios, wheat pasta, and cherries are off limits, you can safely enjoy foods like cucumber, pumpkin seeds, peanuts, quinoa pasta, and cantaloupe. Don't let your mind mess with you! Instead of focusing on the foods you can't have, zero in on the abundance of foods you can enjoy. Your mindset can impact your success, so keep it positive.

Along the way, if you notice there are low FODMAP foods that randomly set you off, remember that just because it's low FODMAP, doesn't mean it's *no* FODMAP. Every food that contains carbs has FODMAPs and even low FODMAP foods eaten in quantities above your body's tolerance level can cause symptoms. That's why rotating foods and eating smaller portions at any given time is also essential to your success. Starting to get the hang of it? I knew you would!

It's important to remember this is a dose-dependent thing. Remember that pot just about to boil over on the stove? You add just a pinch of something and the next thing you know, it's boiling over. The same thing goes for FODMAPs. If your GI system is just about to boil, and you add even a small amount of a high FODMAP food (or low FODMAP food in high amounts), it's game over. It's why one day you can maybe eat an apple, and the next day you can't. It all depends on the dose and how your gut is doing on any given day. This is why it's so important to know your body better!

When you're dealing with a sensitive system, portions really matter. Even if it's a food without FODMAPs (like eggs, olive oil, salmon, or chicken), keep your amounts under control. Be sure to eat every couple of hours and avoid skipping meals. Going for an extended period of time without food can sometimes cause the digestive system to fill up with air, and that alone can cause pain, bloating, and gas.

Also, go slow! Don't lock-and-load your fork. If you've got food in your mouth, chew and swallow before filling up your fork with the next bite. Relax and mindfully enjoy each nourishing bite.

Later on in the book (p. 59-64), I provide you with a list of high and low FODMAP foods. However, please keep this in mind: Foods are still being tested! More foods may prove to be low (*yay!*) and some may be high. If you're going to experiment, use caution. I strongly recommend the Monash University FODMAP Diet App for help with determining which foods are low FODMAP and which ones are high. It's a resource with the most up-to-date information, and the app even includes serving suggestions. It's worth every penny!

When starting with a low FODMAP diet, the number one question I get is: *How long until my symptoms go away?* For some people, the results are immediate, while for others, it can take four to eight weeks (or longer!). You just need to be patient and realize everyone is different. Don't give up.

I've got another important note to share! The symptoms of irritable bowel syndrome (IBS) mimic the symptoms of other "serious" conditions. I say "serious" because as a healthcare provider, any time someone is experiencing symptoms that keep them from living their best life, I take that seriously. But, the good news with IBS is that the condition doesn't cause long-term damage to the body. Unlike celiac disease, gastroesophageal reflux disease (GERD), ulcerative colitis or Crohn's disease (otherwise known as inflammatory bowel disease or IBD), or cancer, IBS irritates but doesn't destroy the GI tract.

It's critical for you to consult with a trusted and caring healthcare provider to make sure your challenging GI issues are not seriously damaging your gut. On that topic, you might find it interesting to know that studies are now showing a reduced FODMAP diet may improve IBD symptoms and GERD, too. So, regardless of your diagnosis, if you've got bloating, gas, diarrhea, constipation, or pain, you could benefit from eating low FODMAP.

---

## BOTTOM LINE

Irrespective of whether you've got an IBS, IBD or GERD diagnosis, if you've got bloating, gas, diarrhea, constipation and/or pain you could benefit from eating low FODMAP.

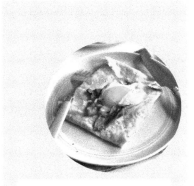

# LOW FODMAP H-I-P DIARY
## Monday

CONTACT

✉ info@thefodmapdoctor.com

🌐 thefodmapdoctor.com

f FODMAP Recipes

♥ FB Group: FODMAP Diet Tips and Support

📷 @thefodmapdoctor

📌 The FODMAP Doctor

## -H-

### {H} HOW YOU FEEL!
Keep track of how you are feeling day by day! Record how you feel physically and emotionally. This will help you to identify potential trigger foods & monitor your progress.

## -I-

### {I} INGREDIENTS!
You've got to know exactly what you're putting into your body! Keep track of each food, and its ingredients. This simple diary can be the key to identifying and eliminating triggers.

## -P-

### {P} PORTION!
Learn the amounts that work for you by keeping track of portion sizes.

### -H-

| | | | |
|---|---|---|---|
| Gas | PERFECT | 0 1 2 3 4 5 6 7 8 9 10 | TERRIBLE |
| Bloating | PERFECT | 0 1 2 3 4 5 6 7 8 9 10 | TERRIBLE |
| Diarrhea | PERFECT | 0 1 2 3 4 5 6 7 8 9 10 | TERRIBLE |
| Constipation | PERFECT | 0 1 2 3 4 5 6 7 8 9 10 | TERRIBLE |
| Abdominal Pain | PERFECT | 0 1 2 3 4 5 6 7 8 9 10 | TERRIBLE |
| Reflux | PERFECT | 0 1 2 3 4 5 6 7 8 9 10 | TERRIBLE |
| Nausea | PERFECT | 0 1 2 3 4 5 6 7 8 9 10 | TERRIBLE |

Mood:

Other:

### -I & P-

Breakfast:

Lunch:

notes

notes

Dinner:

Snacks:

notes

notes

# ELIMINATION PHASE DIET DIARY

During the four to eight weeks of the elimination period, you absolutely must keep track of *everything* you eat and drink. If you experience any symptoms, write it down. Watch for patterns to determine your sensitivities.

When documenting your progress, you want to remember to be HIP!

- ☐ **H: *How you feel*** after eating.

- ☐ **I: *Ingredients*** or the type of food you're eating.

- ☐ **P: *Portion size*** and the amount of food you're eating.

Be really intentional about journaling. I promise this will make all the difference.

## LOW FODMAP GO-TO FOOD IDEAS

There are some days when elaborate recipes are just what I need. For all the other days, what I really need are fast, easy, and healthy meals that I can whip together. Here are a few of my favorite elimination phase go-tos that I know you'll find yourself making over and over again.

### Breakfast:

*Eggs*: I love them scrambled, over easy, sunny-side up, omelette-style, or poached. You can make an egg in under five minutes and eat them in three! Eggs are the perfect way to start the day. I often eat my eggs with a small side of cantaloupe or honeydew melon.

*Gluten-Free Oats*: You can prepare these ahead of time by making overnight oats. All you need is a mason jar, ½ cup of gluten-free rolled oats, and 1 cup of low FODMAP unsweetened milk. I like macadamia milk, but you can also try lactose-free milk, rice, hemp, or almond beverages. You can add in walnuts, ground flax seeds, pecans, peanut butter, pumpkin seeds, chia seeds, blueberries, strawberries, raspberries, spice (like cinnamon, ginger, or nutmeg), and a bit of sweetener (like maple syrup). Add the ingredients to your jar, shake and refrigerate overnight. It's really that simple!

*Cereal with Low FODMAP Milk:* low FODMAP cereal with a splash of milk is a really fast way to start the day. *Recommended brands are listed on my site: thefodmapdoctor.com

*Toast, Tortilla, or Muffin with Peanut Butter and Bananas*: Toast it and top it with all-natural peanut butter, and add a few slices of banana for an on-the-go breakfast.

*Lactose-Free Yogurt*: Look for a lactose-free yogurt that is (ideally) unsweetened. You can sweeten it yourself with fresh berries (just not blackberries!) or a dash of maple syrup. Can't have dairy? Look for coconut-based yogurt alternative.

## Lunch:

*Turkey Burgers*: I prepare these ahead of time so they are ready to go for lunch (or for dinner). I often wrap them in lettuce and add a little mustard.

*Hard-Boiled Eggs*: These are always in our fridge! You can find hard-boiled eggs just about anywhere you go (even when out). These are a fast and easy way to fill up.

*Tuna or Chicken with Pasta*: I mix wild tuna or organic chicken with mayo and gluten-free pasta (usually rice pasta). You can also add in ¼ or less of a medium stalk of diced celery (to either the tuna or chicken salad) or grapes cut in quarters (to the chicken salad).

*Green Salad:* Try a green salad with lettuce, sliced tomato, cucumber, bell peppers, or green beans with a side of whisked olive oil, lemon, salt, and pepper.

*Gluten-Free Bread Sandwich or Tortilla Wrap:* Choose from turkey, roast beef, or baked firm tofu with lettuce, tomato and colby, cheddar, or mozzarella cheese — if you tolerate dairy. If you're a condiment lover (like my husband and kids!), add a touch of mustard or mayo.

## Dinner:

*Baked Salmon with Rice and Pineapple*: I simply bake the salmon with a little salt and pepper until it's firm. Then, I make rice (brown, white, basmati, or wild are all good options), and I serve it with a side of pineapple slices.

*Loaded Baked Potato*: Slice a hot baked potato down the middle and stuff it with your favorite fillings like broccoli (tops only!), cheddar cheese, bacon, tomatoes, or low FODMAP salsa and cilantro.

*Steamed Chicken and Vegetables:* Did you know that most Chinese take-out places offer a dietary version of steamed chicken and veggies with rice? Make sure the order is totally plain (no sauce) and double-check that low FODMAP vegetables like, bok choy, water chestnuts, broccoli tops, carrots, and peppers are included. Ditch the mushrooms, snow peas, or onions. This is totally my go-to take out dinner!

*Quinoa Bowl*: Cook up a bunch of quinoa in advance and make quinoa bowls on the fly! For protein, throw in some eggs, chicken, beef, tofu, or shrimp. Get in a little healthy fat by adding pure olive or sesame oil, pine nuts, walnuts, peanuts, sunflower, or sesame seeds. Get your fruits and veggies in the mix with some kale, broccoli, pineapple, grapes, kiwi, lime, papaya, green beans, bean sprouts, bell peppers, bok choy, carrots, spinach, tomatoes, or zucchini. Soy sauce is low FODMAP (just watch that there's no added sugar or high-fructose corn syrup), and herbs like cilantro, lemongrass, parsley, rosemary, or basil can also add flavor.

## Snacks:

If you don't have a food plan and leave your choices to chance, chances are good those choices will stink! I always (like, always) carry food with me wherever I go. Here are a few of the foods I have ready in my fridge, waiting in my pantry, and packed in my favorite shoulder bag or insulated tote: Clementines, popcorn, carrot sticks, cucumber, pumpkin seeds, bell pepper slices, certified low FODMAP snack bars, macadamia nuts, brazil nuts, walnuts, rice crackers and chips, rice cakes, grapes, and cantaloupe. I also love plain potato crisps, corn chips, gluten-free pretzels (especially with almond butter), and blueberries.

There are also several brands specifically designed for people following a low FODMAP diet! You can find just about everything from soup starters and stocks to ketchup and salsa. *Recommended brands are listed on my site: thefodmapdoctor.com*

Looking for recipes suitable for the elimination phase? Starting on page 68, I've got delicious, easy, simple, and healthy recipes designed with you in mind.

---

### TIP

Don't tolerate a low FODMAP food? Don't over-think it, just don't eat it! You're allowed to be intolerant to a low FODMAP food. It doesn't mean the diet doesn't work, it just means that low FODMAP food doesn't work for you.

*-dr KB*

---

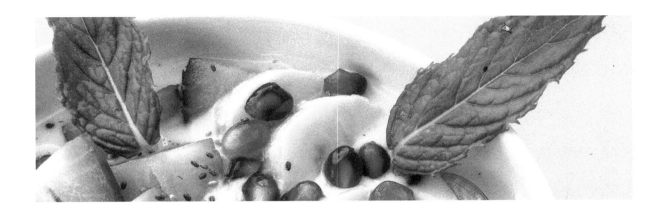

# CHALLENGE PHASE:
# FIGURE IT OUT

Now that you've been eating totally low FODMAP for at least four to eight weeks, you're likely experiencing some real results. I knew you could do it! If you've been sticking to your new diet, you've probably noticed reduced pain, less bloating, decreased GI sensitivity, and better bathroom experiences! Now, let's take it a step further...

Enter: The "Challenge" Phase. Now, here's the part where it really gets interesting — we're going to start incorporating foods higher in FODMAPs, one at a time. Okay, I'm already sensing your hesitation and sweaty palms.

I get it — you're finally feeling better, you're experiencing relief, and now I'm asking you to test the foods you know cause you pain. Take a deep breath, because I'm on your side! This part of the diet is only here to expand the list of foods you can enjoy, so take it slow with me because it will be so worth it.

Aside from incorporating more foods and variety into your diet, experts in the field insist that a strictly low FODMAP diet needs to be challenged. Why? Significantly reducing FODMAPs might affect the bacterial landscape in your intestines. Plus, a lot of foods with high FODMAPs are healthy sources of unique phytonutrients, vitamins, and minerals. It's good to widen the variety of nutrient dense foods in your new diet and work to broaden the list of foods you can tolerate. The goal is to liberalize your dietary restrictions and be healthy. Trust me, don't drive yourself crazy and start stressing over this. Just remember: All you are doing is trying to increase the number and amount of FODMAPs in your intake, so you know what you can tolerate. Let's break it down.

Here's what I've found works best: You're going to challenge each FODMAP for eight days. The groups you'll be challenging are **Galacto-Oligosaccharides** (with either almonds or chickpeas), **Vegetable Fructans** (with onions, garlic, or shallots), **Fruit Fructans** (with raisins, dried dates, or figs), **Grain Fructans** (with spelt or wheat pasta, buckwheat kernels, or couscous), **Bread Fructans** (with bread), **Lactose** (with plain Greek yogurt or milk), **Fructose** (with honey, mango, or sun-dried tomato), **Polyol Mannitol** (with cauliflower, celery, or sweet potato) and the **Polyol Sorbitol** (with avocado or blackberries). Ready to go grocery shopping?

## GET A FOOD SCALE!

Eyeballing the number of ounces in a food is challenging to even a the most nutritiously savvy gal. Remember, it's so important to measure portions when managing FODMAPs.

Each of the foods you'll be incorporating back into your diet only contain one FODMAP. For example, cherries aren't a good challenge food because they contain both fructose and polyols. You wouldn't choose nectarines because they contain both oligos and polyols. If you have a negative reaction to a cherry or a nectarine, it will be harder to detect which FODMAP caused the reaction.

Once you choose your FODMAP food to test, you'll increase the portion size over a three to five day period followed by a three-day washout period (note: you don't need to eat the challenge portion all in one sitting). During the washout period, you'll return to a completely low FODMAP diet and stick to the foods you know are safe for you.

Now, if during the challenge you start experiencing mild symptoms (it might happen!), press on. If the symptoms become strong or too uncomfortable, begin the washout period immediately. You may or may not decide to challenge that group again. But, if you do, perhaps next time try an alternative food from the same group. For example, if onions aren't jiving with your body, you can also challenge garlic. If garlic is still too tough on your body, you can confidently go forward knowing that vegetable fructans are better avoided. It's up to you.

FODMAPs are dose-dependent. So, if you tolerated a low "dose" of avocado, but were set off by a higher "dose," you might want to try again to see how much is too much. A few spoonfuls of guacamole might sit well at the party, but know that eating half of an avocado for breakfast might send you running for the loo.

If you do the entire challenge at once without stopping between testing foods (I don't recommend this), it will last for about eight to 10 weeks. Hang loose, though! Take your time and move through each individual challenge at your own pace. You can choose the order that works the best for you. You've probably already got a sense of which FODMAPs bother you the most.

If in the past, dairy got you down, you might wait to challenge this group last. I also suggest that you challenge your foods on days you don't have anything major going on. If you have an important meeting, family event, or a hot date, you might want to hold off on challenging around those days. If you work outside of your home, you might want to start challenges on a Friday night, or work through them in the evenings to prevent the occurrence of symptoms while at work.

Aside from the one high FODMAP food you've decided to challenge for three to five days, you need to otherwise continue with the low FODMAP diet. Even if you tolerate a high FODMAP food in a previous challenge, for now (the duration of the reintroduction phase), continue to hold off on eating it. A systematic and well-documented approach will be your best chance at long-term accommodation and success. This is the part where you really get to know your body! It's fun!

Reminder: When documenting your progress, you want to be HIP. (p.17)

- ☐ H for **How you feel after eating**
- ☐ I for **Ingredients**
- ☐ P for **Portion Size**

Once you've completed the challenge phase and recorded your results, you'll be more than ready to enter the Reintroduction Phase. This is where we try to put it all together for lasting, long-term relief.

# POLYOLS (SORBITOL)

While you can begin anywhere, I think that the polyols (and avocados in general) are a great place to start. Okay, so here's how it's done: On the first day you'll challenge ¼ of a whole avocado. On the next day you'll test ½ of a whole avocado and on the last day you'll go for one whole avocado. Try to do the challenge over one hour. Don't like avocados? No problem! Test blackberries instead.

- ☐ **Avocado: ¼ (first day), ½ (next day), 1 whole avocado (last day)**

  Wondering what to pair the avocado with? Try adding it to the *Kale, Orange and Feta Salad with Citrus Dressing* (Recipe #13), *Turkey Tacos* (#19), or *Simple Bacon and Egg Salad* (#28).

☐ **Blackberries: 3 (first day), 6 (next day), 10 berries (last day)**

Testing the waters with blackberries instead of avocado? Substitute blackberries for the blueberries in the *Blueberry Fritters* (Recipe #08), try them on top of your *Chia Pudding* (#43) or *Rice Pudding* (#44), add them to your *Fresh Melon Bowl* (#51), or simply toss them into a salad.

If you tolerate **Sorbitol** well, you'll likely be able to eat small portions of apricot, blackberries, cherries, fresh coconut, lychee, nectarine, peach (white or yellow), pears, plum, watermelon, and dried apples, apricots, or prunes in the reintroduction phase and beyond!

---

## 5 HOURS IN SUGAR ALCOHOL HELL

I'm in my early 20s visiting family in Connecticut. My cousin and I are shopping, and in the center of the mall is this huge candy store. At the time, I was in the process of totally changing my approach to food. I completely cut sugar from my diet, and candy was so *not my thing*. But, my cousin was super into it and wanted to fill a little sack with all her faves.

While she's scooping out her Swedish Fish, Charleston Chews, and Fireballs, the sugar-free section of the store catches my eye. I laugh now at my naïve approach, but at the time I had the idea that sugar-free must mean healthy. So, I grabbed a bag, and filled it with sugarless gummy worms and jelly beans. I ate a few while we were walking around and then more on our way home. By the time we walked into the house, I looked 9 months pregnant (no exaggeration) and was in *excruciating* pain. I literally couldn't bear it. I crawled up in a ball next to the bathroom and felt like I had journeyed down a rabbit hole into gastrointestinal hell. My family was debating what to do and was thinking about calling an ambulance, but I resisted. To this day, I am so happy I did. They would have diagnosed me with gas pain. Ugh. Gas pain. As it was, the whole experience was embarrassing enough without a trip to the emergency room. Needless to say, the horrific pain continued for hours until at last, my body (in a relatively violent fashion), eliminated the offending polyols. So not cool!

It wasn't until years later when I started to understand the effects of sugar alcohols, that I understood what happened to me. I realize now that the sugar-free candy I ate was loaded up with polyols (otherwise known as sugar alcohols) like sorbitol, mannitol, xylitol, maltitol, maltitol syrup, lactitol, erythritol, isomalt, and hydrogenated starch hydrolysate. For a person who is sensitive to FODMAPs, sugar free (polyol-full) "treats" are really a one way ticket down the GI rabbit hole into the abyss of pain, bloating, and bathroom explosion. For this reason, even if you test okay for polyols, I *strongly* recommend completely avoiding any kind of sugar-free processed food. Also, always read the list of ingredients on your labels and steer clear of sugar alcohols.

# POLYOLS (MANNITOL)

You can test polyols a few different ways. You can try cauliflower, celery, or sweet potato. I recommend going with sweet potato first. You only have to challenge one, but I find that testing a few is even more beneficial. Here are the amounts you want to go with for the three days of your challenge:

☐ **Cauliflower: 1 oz. (first day), 2 oz. (next day), 3 oz. (last day)**

> You can roast the cauliflower along with your *Fingerling Potatoes* (Recipe #33), try it steamed, add it to the *Beef with Broccoli* (#26), toss it in a salad or enjoy cauliflower rice. To make cauliflower rice, all you have to do is grate it with a hand-grater or food processor, then sauté it in a large pan with a little olive oil and salt. Cover the "rice" for a few minutes to let it steam.

☐ **Celery: ½ (first day), 1 (next day), 2 whole sticks (last day)**

> Try adding chopped celery to your *Wild Rice, Zucchini, Fennel and Walnuts* (Recipe #25), *Chicken and Wild Rice Soup* (#17), *Easy Wok Vegetables* (#34), or *Pineapple and Cucumber Salad* (#36). You might also enjoy celery with nut butter.

☐ **Sweet Potato: 3 oz. (first day), 5 oz. (next day), 7 oz. (last day)**

> Baked or roasted, sweet potato is delicious. Try baked sweet potato with cinnamon or roasted sweet potatoes with parsnips. You can substitute sweet potatoes for white potatoes in your *Perfect Potatoes* (Recipe #31) or *Potato Chips* (#39).

If you tolerate **Mannitol** well, once you're in the reintroduction phase, you'll likely be able to eat small portions of butternut squash, mushrooms (shiitake, portobello, button), snow peas, and pumpkin.

# GALACTO-OLIGOSACCHARIDES (GOS/OLIGOS)

If you're a vegan or vegetarian with irritable bowel symptoms, chances are you've struggled to steer clear of GOS foods during the elimination phase of the diet. Galacto-oligosaccharides are chains of galactose that are commonly found in a lot of the most common vegan and vegetarian sources of protein, like nuts, and beans. When challenging GOS foods, pick from either almonds or chickpeas.

- ☐ **Almonds: 15 (first day), 20 (next day), 25 almonds (last day)**

    Almonds are a perfect addition to the *Pineapple Rice* (Recipe #32), *Easy Wok Vegetables* (#34), *Cocoa Banana Smoothie* (#48) or the *Spiced Nuts* (#50). Or, you can try substitute almonds for pecans in the *Orange Pecan Granola* (#09), or for the walnuts in the *Wild Rice with Zucchini, Fennel, & Walnuts* (#25).

- ☐ **Canned Chickpeas: ½ (first day), ⅔ (next day), 1 cup (last day)**

    Chickpeas are perfect to use for a quick addition to any green salad (try mixed greens, with beans, grilled chicken or shrimp, tomato, cucumber, oil, and lemon). You can also try serving them on top of the *Chicken and Wild Rice Soup* (Recipe #17) or the *Gazpacho* (#27).

If you tolerate **GOS/Oligos** well, once you're in the reintroduction phase, you'll likely be able to eat small portions of cashews, hazelnuts, pistachios, haricot beans, lima beans, and green peas.

# FRUCTANS

Fructans are a group of carbohydrates commonly found in bread, vegetables, fruit, and processed foods. Your body has a hard time breaking down fructans because you (*and everyone else*) lack the enzymes needed to break carbohydrate chains. Additionally, only about 5-15% of fructans are absorbed in the small intestine, which means they are passed into the large intestine where they are fermented. The leftover particles draw lots of water into the large intestine, setting the stage for lots of gas and diarrhea. Due to varying chemical structures found in these foods, I think it's important to test fructan groups one at a time. It's why you'll challenge vegetable, fruit, grain, and bread fructans separately.

## VEGETABLE FRUCTANS

- ☐ **Spanish Onions: ¼ (first day), ½ (next day), 1 whole onion (last day)**
    Test with Spanish Onions as white onion may contain GOS in higher amounts.

- ☐ **Garlic: ¼ (first day), ½ (next day), 1 whole clove (last day)**

- ☐ **Shallots: ½ (first day), 1 (next day), 2 whole shallots (last day)**

As a general rule, unless you really love them raw, I suggest you don't eat onions, garlic or shallots uncooked. Try them roasted or sautéed instead. You can add these flavorful foods to almost any dish.

If you tolerate **Vegetable Fructans** well, you likely can handle small amounts of artichoke, beetroot, leek, button mushrooms, and snow peas in the reintroduction phase.

# FRUIT FRUCTANS

☐ **Raisins: 1 tbsp. (first day), 2 tbsp. (next day), 4 tbsp. (last day)**

You can eat raisins alone, mix them with peanuts, or try adding them to the *Orange Pecan Granola* (Recipe #09), the *Oh-So-Good Oatmeal* (#03), the *Kale, Orange, & Feta Salad with Citrus Dressing* (#13), the *Chicken Pecan Grape Salad Sandwich* (#14), or the *Broccoli and Bacon Salad* (#30).

☐ **Dried Dates: 1 (first day), 2 (next day), 4 whole dates (last day)**

Dates naturally sweeten up smoothies. You might enjoy adding dates to the *Morning Glory Smoothie* (#04). And when chopped, they pair nicely with nuts, granola, and oatmeal.

If you tolerate **Fruit Fructans** well, you can try small amounts of apricots (fresh or dried), super ripe bananas, grapefruit, nectarines, peaches, plums, pomegranate, watermelon, figs, mango, and prunes in the reintroduction phase.

# GRAIN FRUCTANS

*If you have celiac disease do NOT test gluten-containing grains. The only acceptable grain to test or otherwise eat is buckwheat, which doesn't contain gluten.

☐ **Spelt or Wheat Pasta: 3 oz. (first day), 5 oz. (next day), 7 oz. (last day)**

Try substituting wheat noodles for the rice noodles in the *Stir Fried Shrimp and Rice Noodles* (Recipe #11) recipe or replace the zucchini with noodles in the *Veggie Noodles with Pesto and Cherry Tomato* (#20). Instead of using gluten-free pasta, you can use wheat or spelt pasta in the *Rotini Pasta with Cherry Tomato and Arugula* (#15) or the *Roasted Red Peppers with Tomato Sauce and Pasta* (#23).

☐ **Buckwheat Kernels: 2 oz. (first day), 3 oz. (next day), 5 oz. (last day)**

Buckwheat kernels are sometimes also referred to as Kasha. You can make Kasha into a breakfast cereal (and serve with banana slices, almond milk, and maple syrup) or into a savory side dish (substitute for brown rice). Try substituting buckwheat for rice in the *Wild Rice, Zucchini, Fennel and Walnuts* (Recipe #25) recipe.

Feeling good with **Grain Fructans**? You'll probably be fine with wheat bran, barley, rye, couscous, freekeh, and wheat germ in the reintroduction phase.

## GLUTEN SENSITIVITY WITHOUT CELIAC? IT'S PROBABLY THE FRUCTANS.

Have you ever noticed that gluten-free eating might relieve discomfort, even if you've tested negative for celiac disease? Chances are it's not the protein (gliadin) in wheat or gluten-containing grains that you're reacting to, but rather the carbohydrates called fructans that are at the root of your symptoms. A celiac diagnosis means no gluten again, ever, for life. If you only have an issue with fructans, though, you may still be able to tolerate gluten-containing foods in smaller amounts.

## BREAD FRUCTANS

☐ **Wheat Bread 1 (first day), 2 (next day), 3 slices (last day)**

If you've got celiac disease or a known gluten sensitivity, you're going to just skip this challenge. Otherwise, you can try bread toasted with a spread of nut butter and sliced banana, with the *Chicken Pecan Grape Salad Sandwich* (Recipe #14), in the *Banana French Toast* (#01) or served with soup. Remember this: You don't need to eat the challenge portion all in one sitting.

# LACTOSE

Lactose is especially tricky, even for people without a sensitive digestive system. It's a real challenge for a lot of people, since our bodies are generally limited in the ability to make lactase (the enzyme that breaks down lactose). The older you get, the less lactase your body makes. It's why lactose intolerance is so common! If you already know you are lactose intolerant or just feel like dairy doesn't do it for you, you can skip this challenge.

☐ **Organic Plain Greek Yogurt: 2 oz. (first day), 4 oz. (next day), 8 oz. (last day)**

Greek Yogurt is delicious and loaded with protein. For general health and wellness, I recommend the organic variety without sugar. Greek yogurt pairs perfectly with *Orange Pecan Granola* (Recipe #09). You can also substitute the lactose-free yogurt with Greek yogurt in the *Yogurt Parfait Recipe* (#10) or simply eat it with a little low FODMAP fruit and a drizzle of maple syrup for sweetness.

☐ **Cow's Milk: 3 oz. (first day), 5 oz. (next day), 8 oz. (last day)**

Enjoy some milk with your favorite low FODMAP cereal or *Orange Pecan Granola* (#49). You can also try some milk and *Oatmeal Cookies* (#49) or *Biscotti* (#52).

# FRUCTOSE

You'll likely always need to monitor the amount of fructose (fruit sugar) you consume at any one time. Lots of gals who are sensitive to FODMAPs are also just generally overly sensitive to fructose.

☐ **Honey: 1 tsp. (first day), 1 tbsp. (next day), 2 tbsp. (last day)**

I love adding honey to my gluten-free oatmeal, lactose-free yogurt and favorite baked goods. You can replace the maple syrup with honey in the *No Bake Peanut Butter Balls* (Recipe #46), *Rice Pudding* (#44), *Lemonade* (#53), *Oatmeal Cookies* (#49), *Chia Pudding* (#43), and *Rice Treats* (#47).

☐ **Mango: ¼ (first day), ½ (next day), 1 whole fruit (last day)**

Add mangos to your *Strawberry Kiwi Banana Pops* (Recipe #45), replace the pineapple with mango in the *Morning Glory Smoothie* (#04) and the *Pineapple Rice* (#32) or add it to the *Fresh Melon Bowl* (#51). Or try my family's all time favorite dessert, frozen mangos.

☐ **Sun-Dried Tomato: 4 (first day), 8 (next day), 12 pieces (last day)**

Sun-dried tomatoes are awesome in pasta and salads. They would make the perfect addition to *Rotini Pasta with Cherry Tomato and Arugula* (Recipe #15) or the *Tomato Basil Millet* (#29).

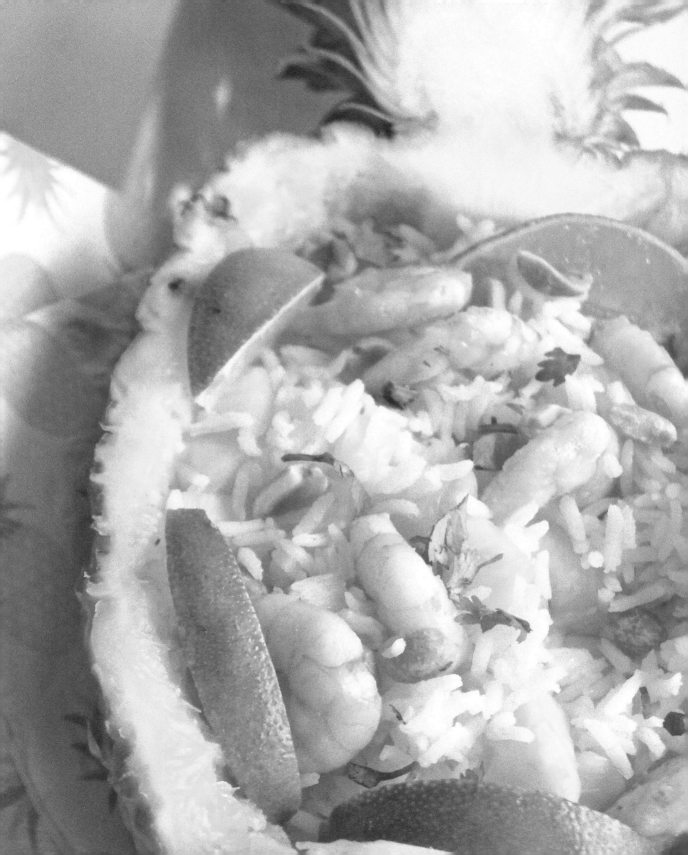

# TIPS:

☐ It doesn't really matter if you eat the challenge food cooked or raw. But, I would say that you should stick with the method you initially choose throughout the challenge. For example, if you're testing vegetable fructans with onion and you choose to have a stir fry on the first day of the challenge, don't go for raw onions on the second day.

☐ Don't eat a challenge food by itself. The sheer act of eating a high FODMAP food on an "empty" stomach could cause bloating and other symptoms. Eat your challenge food with a typical low FODMAP meal so your body has an easier time digesting it.

☐ Be determined and stay positive even when your results are a bummer. Let's say you love and miss milk, yet when you challenge lactose, you live in the bathroom for two days. Even though you can't have dairy for now, doesn't mean you'll never have dairy again. You can always challenge it again down the road.

☐ Sometimes, reactions are immediate, while others might take a day or two. Be mindful that a reaction to a challenge food may be delayed.

☐ Stress and hormones (*Hello, period belly!*) or even foodborne bacteria (like E. coli or salmonella) can affect your system. Realize that while most of the time it's FODMAPs, sometimes other factors are confounding. Don't give up!

☐ Once you've challenged each group, you can feel pretty comfortable about your tolerance levels. For example, if you challenged sweet potato (mannitol) at five ounces, you should probably be fine with a typical two-ounce serving of cauliflower (also mannitol). What about with honey and mangos (fructose)? Or polyols, like sweet potato and avocado? If you were able to handle those food items, you will likely be fine with a small amount of cherries (which are high in polyols, plus fructose).

☐ Avoid portion distortion. Stick to the recommended portions for each FODMAP challenge while continuing to eat small portions in general. Think more mini-meals (never mega-meals). As a general rule, I recommend six mini-meals a day, rather than three large ones.

# REACTION SURVIVAL KIT

**Here's how to deal.** First and foremost, don't be surprised and don't get freaked out if you have a negative reaction to a high FODMAP food. And by the way, it's normal to face some sort of reaction along the way. Take a deep breath — a low and slow deep abdominal breath. Breathe in for a slow count of four and out for an even slower count of six. Do this 10 times. Remind yourself that to some extent, setbacks are inevitable, and you can and *will* be able to deal with it.

Next, get out your measuring cup and keep yourself hydrated! Did you know that you should be drinking at least half of your bodyweight in ounces? So, if you weigh 200 pounds, you need a minimum of 100 ounces of water. Hydrate, hydrate, hydrate! Drink small amounts throughout the day — don't start guzzling at night to meet that goal. Also, keep this in mind: Some people just don't tolerate water well within an hour of eating. One more thing? Cold water with a hot meal or hot water with a cold meal can sometimes be a trigger for sensitive individuals.

If bloating, gas, and pain are on the attack, fight back with a couple of yoga poses. Start on your back for the "Wind-Relieving Pose" otherwise known as Apanasana. Deeply inhale and place your hands on your knees. Hug your knees up to your chest as you gently exhale. Exhale, and hug your knees to your chest. If it's comfortable, maintain this position (lying on your back with your knees pulled into your chest) and rock gently from side to side. Stay in the position while connecting with your breath for about one minute. Relax as you lower the soles of your feet back to the floor and repeat as needed.

Another go-to yoga pose is the famous child's pose, otherwise known as Balasana. First, place a pillow in front of you. Next, sit on your knees about two feet behind the pillow with your shins to the floor. Leave a little space between each leg. Slowly, lean forward and stretch your arms out in front of you. Then, keeping your back straight, place your forehead gently onto the pillow. Take a few deep breaths. If you find these poses to be helpful and effective, look up and try other alternatives such as the Cat and Cow (otherwise known as Marjaryasana and Bitilasana) or the Downward-Facing Dog (otherwise known as Adho Mukha Savanasana).

A heating pad or hot pack, abdominal massage, and light exercise are also great options for decreasing discomfort. Apply a hot pack to your abdomen for about 15 minutes every hour as needed. When massaging, take a little bit of lotion or cream (I prefer unscented) and rub your abdomen clockwise — start from the outer edges of your abdomen and work your way in towards the belly button with concentric circles. For exercise, just do what feels best for you! Try to aim for at least 20 minutes of movement each day. Even a walk around your neighborhood will do you good!

Make a list of go-to foods that you know are totally okay for your gut. This way if (when) you flare up, you'll be able to go right back to the basics and get yourself feeling better.

I've noticed (both personally and professionally) that foods like chicken, salmon, turkey, rice, cucumbers, cantaloupe, eggs, baked potato, pumpkin seeds, rice noodles, and gluten-free oatmeal (with maple syrup) seem to settle the issue.

This is the time to treat yourself very kindly. As you're learning more about your body, connecting with it, and the foods you eat, you've got to be patient and practice some self-love. Schedule in things you love to do. Keep your mind more on the life you want to live than the foods you want to eat. Schedule in some good (non-food related) rewards after each challenge. Got through the fructans? Get a pedicure! Lived through lactose? Buy tickets for a fun movie, concert, or show. Managed the polyols? Go get a massage! Do whatever you need to do to keep your attitude elevated.

## NOT EXPERIENCING RELIEF? DON'T PANIC!

You may need to continue the elimination phase for a few more weeks and make sure you assess whether or not you are strictly sticking to your new diet. Research shows that one in four sufferers don't experience total relief with the diet, though it's commonly thought that the reason is simply because they aren't following the diet closely enough to make a real difference.

If you've been strict about sticking to your diet and you're still not finding relief, this might be the time to involve a professional who specializes in FODMAP nutrition. Keep in mind, it's okay to have more than one thing go wrong in your body at the same time. So, if you're not noticing an improvement after six weeks, make it a priority to consult with a doctor you trust.

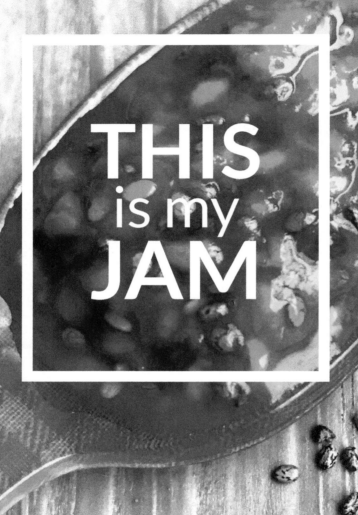

THIS
is my
JAM

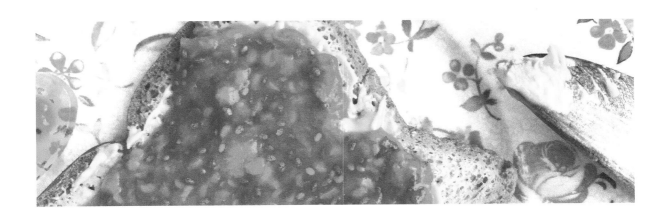

# REINTRODUCTION PHASE: LEARN TO LIVE WITH IT

Get excited, because now the experiment really begins. You're going to turn yourself into a guinea pig (they're so cute, just like you!) and work towards broadening the scope of your diet in a significant way. I think a key to long-term success involves keeping a diary. At least for now, you've got to keep tracking what you eat and how you feel to fully heal. Remember, there are three "HIP" aspects of your new diet that you need to record how you feel, ingredients, and portion (p.17).

Now that you've challenged your groups (galacto-oligosaccharides, vegetable fructans, fruit fructans, grain fructans, bread fructans, fructose, mannitol, and sorbitol) and have a feel for which ones *and* which amounts are the best for your body, you can start slowly reintroducing a combination of higher FODMAP foods into your everyday diet. Reminder, if at any time you experience a setback, all you've got to do is practice a low FODMAP "washout" for two to three days to get yourself back on track. Don't stress it. You're going to be okay!

**I created for you a list of foods broken down by specific FODMAP type. You can use it as a reference and guide...**

# HIGH FODMAP FOODS BY FODMAP TYPE

## GALACTO-OLIGOSACCHARIDES (GOS/OLIGOS)

- [ ] Almonds
- [ ] Black Beans
- [ ] Cashews
- [ ] Chickpeas
- [ ] Green Peas
- [ ] Haricot Beans
- [ ] Hazelnut
- [ ] Lima Beans
- [ ] Pistachio
- [ ] Red Kidney Beans
- [ ] Savoy Cabbage

## FRUCTANS (VEGETABLE)

- [ ] Artichoke
- [ ] Beetroot
- [ ] Button Mushrooms
- [ ] Garlic
- [ ] Green Onions and Scallion bulbs
- [ ] Leek
- [ ] Snow Peas
- [ ] Spanish Onions
- [ ] White Onion

## FRUCTANS (GRAINS)

- [ ] Barley
- [ ] Buckwheat Kernels
- [ ] Couscous
- [ ] Freekeh
- [ ] Rye
- [ ] Sprouted Wheat Grain
- [ ] Wheat
- [ ] Wheat Bran
- [ ] Wheat Germ
- [ ] Wheat Noodles and Pasta

## FRUCTANS (FRUIT)

- [ ] Apricots
- [ ] Banana, overly ripe
- [ ] Dates
- [ ] Dried Apricot
- [ ] Dried Figs
- [ ] Dried Mango
- [ ] Grapefruit
- [ ] Nectarine
- [ ] Plum
- [ ] Pomegranate
- [ ] Prunes
- [ ] Watermelon
- [ ] White Peaches

## FRUCTANS (BREAD)

- [ ] Multigrain Bread
- [ ] Wheat Bread
- [ ] White Bread

## LACTOSE

- [ ] Buttermilk
- [ ] Cream Cheese
- [ ] Custard
- [ ] Haloumi Cheese
- [ ] Ice Cream
- [ ] Kefir
- [ ] Milk
- [ ] Sour Cream
- [ ] Yogurt

## FRUCTOSE

- [ ] Apples
- [ ] Asparagus
- [ ] Boysenberry
- [ ] Broccolini
- [ ] Cherries
- [ ] Dark and Light Agave Syrup

- [ ] Dried Apples
- [ ] Dried Pears
- [ ] Feijoa
- [ ] Honey
- [ ] Mango
- [ ] Pears
- [ ] Sugar Snap Peas
- [ ] Sultanas
- [ ] Sun-Dried Tomatoes
- [ ] Unripe Guava
- [ ] Watermelon
- [ ] Broccoli Stalks

## POLYOLS (MANNITOL)

- [ ] Butternut Squash
- [ ] Celery
- [ ] Mushrooms: Portobello, Shiitake, and Button
- [ ] Pumpkin
- [ ] Snow Peas

## POLYOLS (SORBITOL)

- [ ] Apples
- [ ] Apricot
- [ ] Avocado
- [ ] Blackberries
- [ ] Cherries
- [ ] Dried Apples
- [ ] Dried Apricots
- [ ] Fresh Coconut
- [ ] Longan
- [ ] Lychee
- [ ] Nectarine
- [ ] Peaches
- [ ] Pears
- [ ] Plum
- [ ] Prunes
- [ ] Watermelon

Just like the challenge phase, in the reintroduction phase, you'll need to be systematic. While in the challenge phase, your focus was figuring out which FODMAP groups work the best for you, in the reintroduction phase, you'll determine the cumulative effect of FODMAPs in your everyday diet. Phew, let me explain...

If you eat all low FODMAP foods for breakfast (eggs, cantaloupe, and potatoes) what you're trying to figure out is how much of a total FODMAP load you can tolerate for the rest of the day so you're not a bloated mess by the time 5:00 rolls around. For example, if the oligo, mannitol, and fructose groups went well during the challenge phase, now you want to see what happens when you eat a salad with pistachios (oligos), celery (mannitol), and fresh figs (fructose) for lunch and a bowl of garlic (oligos) chicken with mango (fructose) rice. You're figuring out the right load of FODMAPs that works for you. The best way to do this is to document every food experience until you feel totally comfortable and have your symptoms well under control. You'll be like a natural in no time.

When you're keeping track of symptoms, it's best to use a Borg Pain Scale — a fancy term for rating your symptoms on a scale of one to ten. A rating of one means you are symptom-free, and a rating of ten means it's beyond what you can bear. Next, you need to determine what's tolerable for you. For example, if you really love eating apples, and you know eating one causes your abdomen to bloat and a level of pain you'd rate a two out of ten, you might decide the apple is worth it. But, if two apples in one day puts you at a pain level of six out of ten, you might feel like that's not justifiable. It's all about *your* tolerance of the dose. It's all about you!

The whole reintroduction phase is really all about you getting to know yourself. The goal is to *know* what food combinations work best for your body and *grow* in the confidence of your food choices. Once you know what works, you'll fearlessly eat the foods that you like and make you feel good.

And remember, this is an ongoing process. Digestive issues are not like the common cold or a virus where you've got it for a few weeks — and then you don't. Likely, you're going to be dealing with some extent of symptoms for awhile. You've got to choose to live #FODMAPfabulous. Own your style of eating like a boss! Don't let your "diet" drag you down, instead use food as a way to rise. Rise above the pain and live the life you've always imagined.

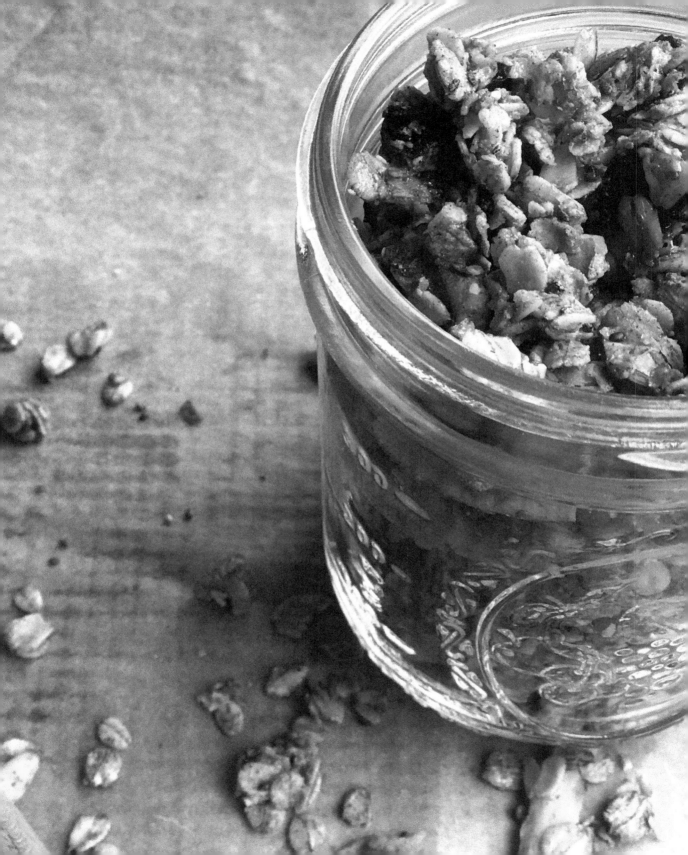

Sometimes the same ingredient can be low or high FODMAP depending on how it's processed. If this is confusing you, you're not alone! The fermentability and chemical structure of any given food can vary depending on how it's processed. That's why coconut water, fresh coconut, and coconut flour are high FODMAP while dried coconut, coconut oil, coconut milk, coconut sugar and coconut yogurt are all low FODMAP. Hang in there! It will become second nature soon enough.

## Eat a wide variety of foods

Once you find a few foods you know you can safely eat (that also taste good), you probably will want to eat them over and over again. Been there, done that? I want to inspire you to incorporate a variety of foods into your diet and encourage you to not limit yourself.

When you eat the same foods all the time, you limit the types of nutrients coming into your body. Every real and whole food (food that comes from the earth, not from a test tube) contains different kinds of nutrients like vitamins, minerals, phytochemicals, and antioxidants. These nutrients work together in synergy to enable your body to prevent and fight disease. Variety really is key to overall health!

Just remember, almost every food, (even very healthy food) carries some risk. There's arsenic in rice, PCBs and dioxins in fish, oxalates in spinach, pesticides on produce, aflatoxins found on peanuts, GMOs with corn, and the list goes on.

But take heart! You were born with an amazing detox system. A generally healthy body is more than capable of eliminating what's not good and keeping what's needed. This is why it's important that you don't eat the same foods over and over again and stress your system with the same toxins.

By rotating the foods in your diet, you'll protect your detox system from overload while giving your body the nutrients it needs. Eat a variety of foods in smaller portions and your body will thank you for the added protection.

## BOTTOM LINE

As you work through your reintroduction phase, keep this in mind — It's important to try to liberalize your diet the best you can, but the ultimate goal is long-term pain and symptom reduction. The single most important thing is eating so you feel good!

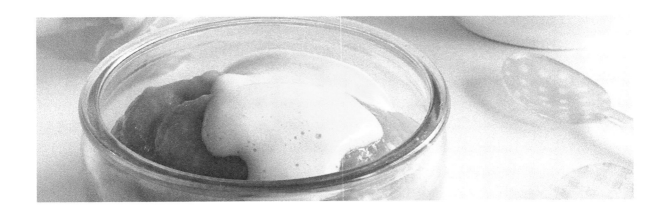

# WHAT TO EAT WHEN EATING OUT

When it comes to eating low FODMAP-style, eating out might feel totally overwhelming. You're more or less at the mercy of a string of people making, plating, and serving your food. And if you're eating out, it's likely you're not alone. Chances are good that you're "enjoying" a meal out with friends or at a family event — so, spending the time looking like you're seven months pregnant or spending an hour in the bathroom isn't an option.

You've got a couple of ways to deal with this, so let's first discuss restaurants. If you know where you'll be eating, I recommend scoping out the menu online or reaching out to the eatery in advance to see which options are available to you. If your group is making dinner plans, you can always recommend the places you've had a positive experience at. Remember, stress can also trigger symptoms, so the less stress going into a meal, the better. Just keep in mind, no matter where you dine, you'll always be the one in total control of what goes into your mouth!

If it's a place that's totally new to you, you might want to consider eating something before you go. I know, it's not sexy, but it works. Then, you just order a simple salad with lettuce, tomato, cucumber, olive oil, and lemon (or something else you are confident is low FODMAP and easy for the chef to execute) and simply enjoy the company free of anxiety.

If the menu isn't conducive to your new style of eating, that doesn't mean you have to sit there experiencing #FOMO while the rest of your party chows down. If you're feeling a bit brave or are really just feeling hungry, it's worth a quick talk with the manager. You can discreetly visit the hostess stand and request a quick chat with the manager. Just be direct about what you'd like to eat and how it needs to be prepared. He or she will give you an honest assessment of whether or not the kitchen can make that work, and as a bonus, will likely personally manage the order.

Let's say the order doesn't come out right. It's frustrating, but just don't eat it. If you think it's worth ordering again, go for it. But if it seems like it's too much of a pain, just count it as a loss. I know the temptation is there to avoid the questions and comments from onlookers, but feeling sick just isn't worth it. When in doubt, give it to someone else at your table or send it back. It's better in the trash than trashing your body. Now is the time to release any guilt you may feel about getting rid of a plate you know will make you sick.

Do you ever feel funky about the way other people view your eating habits? Trust me, the less awkward you appear, the less awkward others will feel. Be confident (or just fake it 'til you make it) about your food choices and style of eating. The more you own it, the less it will own you. If you make a big deal about it, complain about it, and bemoan it, you'll draw negative attention to yourself and your condition. If you act positive and like it's no big deal, it won't be. You're living in a modern age where gluten-free, dairy-free, paleo, vegan, AIP, no added sugar, and other "special" diets reign. So, put your crown on and own your style of eating as the best choice for you body — others will respect it and respect you for it.

Don't feel like explaining FODMAPs and your issues with gas, bloating, and diarrhea to the person you're dining with? No problem. All you have to do is be direct. Simply say, "I am working on improving my health with a diet recommended by my doctor." That's it. Case closed! They keep pushing for details? Redirect the conversation by asking about their kids, work, hobbies, or the weather. Never feel like you need to excuse, defend, or explain your food choices. You're doing this for you because it's what's best for your body. End of story.

Now, let's say you're eating out at a party, event, or someone else's home. If you're close to the person, offer to bring food (appetizer, entree, or dessert) and bring dishes that you know work for your diet. I've got plenty of recipe ideas for you to choose from! You can also just let the host know you're on a special diet for medical reasons and bring along your own food. Another option is to just eat before you go and leave a little easy-to-eat snack in your bag. I often carry clementines and pumpkin seeds along with me. They're filling, easy to carry, easy to eat, and a little sweet!

Okay, now let's talk about food-pushers. There's always at least one in every group. You know, the person who can't take the fact that you aren't eating the pizza or trying a piece of cake? Dealing with food-pushers can at times be a real challenge — some people just *do not get it*. They won't take no for an answer! Even though their intentions are good, it can be so uncomfortable to deal with their incessant and relentless need to feed you foods that will undoubtedly make you miserable. If you've got a close relationship with the food-pusher, make a time (preferably before the next event) to privately discuss your issue and politely ask that they stop pushing. They might not even realize they're doing it. If it's someone you're not really close to, be firm, direct, and simply answer, "No thanks!" every time they ask. If you stay strong, most of the time they generally do back down and eventually move on (and look for a weaker target).

Here's the bottom line and major takeaway: You'll get so much more from your eating out experience when you focus more on the relationships you have with the people you are dining with than focusing on your relationship with food. Food comes and goes. But hopefully the relationships you cultivate around the table will last a lifetime. Focus on what really matters, and you'll leave the experience feeling full and satisfied in every sense.

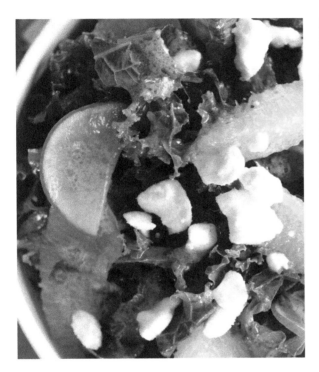 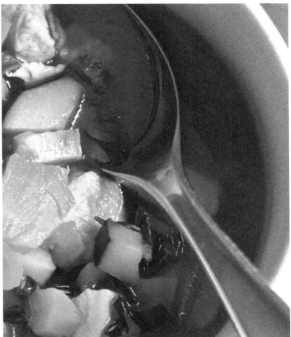

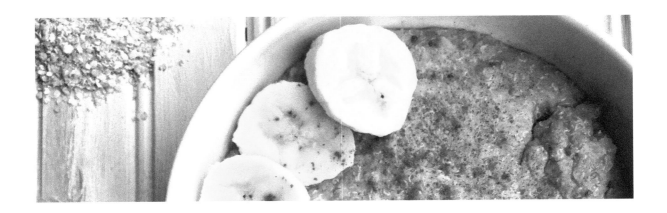

# MAKE IT WORK: PLAN YOUR MEALS

You've got a delicious opportunity to get your body working for you again. I get messages and emails from people around the world (literally) who've been instructed by their doctor or health practitioner to begin a low FODMAP diet. All too often, they're confident this dietary prescription is a culinary death sentence and start fearing eating rice cakes and peanut butter for the rest of their lives. This is so not the case. Open your eyes, your heart, and your mind to the possibilities! Adjust your attitude. There are so many combinations of foods that can taste great and be great for you. You've got to figure out how to get those combinations working for you. Let's talk logistics.

> ### TIP
>
> If you have a few favorite go-to meals, try to find alternative ways to prepare them. If your favorite food is impossible to recreate, become intentional about finding new foods that you love. Mindset matters!
>
> *—dr KB*

*If you don't have a plan and leave your choices to chance, chances are good, your choices will stink.* I think that having a plan in place, whether it be a specific meal plan, a routine you stick to weekly, or a month-long gameplan for what you'll be eating is key. You've essentially got three choices on how to approach your food strategy:

☐ **Stick with a week-long meal plan that includes breakfast, lunch, and dinner with room for snacks after each meal:**

Since I began practicing over a decade ago, I have been creating these types of plans. This strategy is great for people who are very structured and like things completely planned out. If you think this type of strategy might work well for you, I offer a meal plan option on my website www.thefodmapdoctor.com

☐ **Keep only low FODMAP foods in your fridge, pantry, and freezer:**

Prep, make, and eat whatever, whenever. This approach will be a good one if you're super laid back and easy going. If you like your world unstructured, this food prep style is best for you.

☐ **Get into a food routine. In other words, pick certain meal genres for certain days:**

This is the strategy that works best for me. This way, I'm in a routine — but never in a rut. I have a general idea of what I'll be making but have flexibility in how I'll make it. In our house, Mondays are for oatmeal, sandwiches, and something meatless. Tuesdays are for cereal, salad, and tacos. Wednesdays are all about waffles with smoothies, soups, and breakfast for dinner. Thursdays we enjoy muffins, fish, and pasta. On Fridays we do eggs, grain bowls, and pizza. Saturdays are the best days, because we start with french toast, heat up some leftovers for lunch, and end with turkey or fish burgers. Then Sundays, we usually have crepes for brunch and stir-fry for supper.

Hate recording what you eat and feel like? Then, unless you're figuring it out in the challenge phase, don't. For most people keeping a food diary works, but for others, a long-term commitment to a diet journal might feel unnatural and drive them crazy. If it's making you crazy, just give it a rest. Start easing into a low FODMAP life without all of the writing by tuning in to your body's signals. Focus on intuitive eating for a week or so and see how that works for you.

# ASK YOURSELF THESE THREE QUESTIONS:

*Is my need for this food a craving?* Generally, food cravings are a sign of emotional hunger. If you're craving kale it's completely possible that you are experiencing true hunger, but if it's a candy bar, chips, or a cookie you're after, it's likely that you are eating to satisfy an emotion with a burst of pleasure. When you're truly hungry, almost any food will suffice.

*Is there a rumbling?* When you have a healthy relationship with food, your body will signal for more nutrients with physical sensations (like a rumbling in the stomach). However, for many emotional eaters, the physical sensations of hunger are overridden by food desires.

*When did I last eat?* True hunger generally presents itself at regular intervals. If you've recently eaten, chances are good you don't need that food in front of you. When you're eating emotionally, it doesn't matter whether or not you are full. True hunger can be satisfied with a healthy meal. Emotionally hunger is never satisfied.

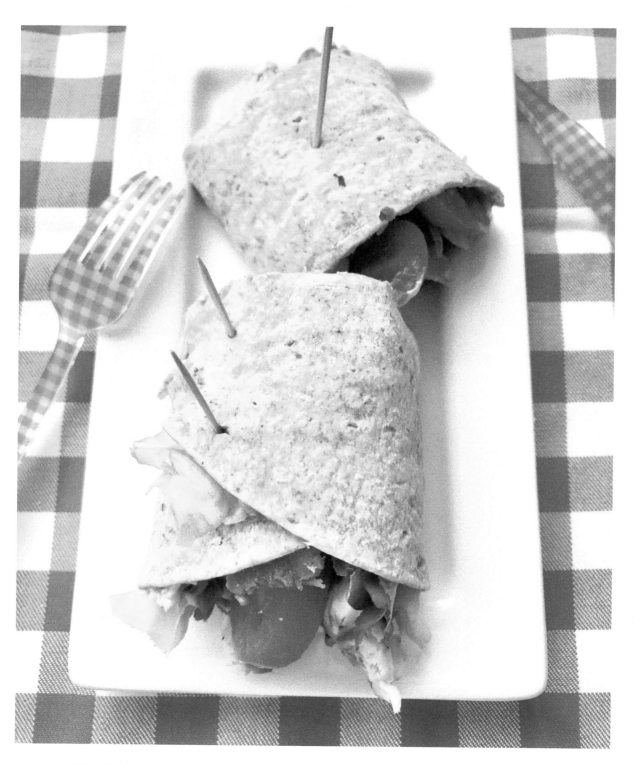

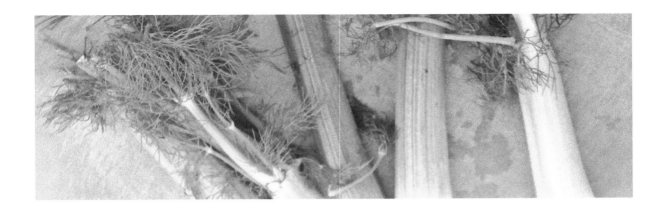

# HOW TO PREPARE YOUR MEALS

If you've never really liked spending time in the kitchen and aren't even quite sure which end of the knife is sharp (wink), this section is for you. I've found that most of the cool gals who are getting started don't have time to spend hours on food prep. So, here's the deal—keep it easy. My food prep philosophy is pretty simple: Combine low FODMAP ingredients, keep 'em raw (when appropriate) or heat them up (when it's better that way), throw in "safe" spices (like salt, pepper, basil, thyme, rosemary, cinnamon, ginger, turmeric, paprika, parsley, or tarragon) and eat. Focus on easy cooking styles that fit into your schedule and work for you and the people you live with!

## GRILLING

Grilling is a great way to prepare meats, fruit, and veggies fast with minimal prep or clean up. While I love it, I'm careful about the way I grill. When you grill meat, there's a risk that you might be creating and eating some cancer-causing agents — you know, carcinogens. The best way to keep your grilling healthy is to simply prepare your meat with an antioxidant-rich marinade. To make the marinade, start by choosing an oil with a high smoke point such as organic canola oil, avocado oil, or pure olive oil. You'll need about ½ cup of oil per pound of meat, and for fish, a little less. Next, whisk in your favorite herbs like rosemary, turmeric, basil, oregano, sage, parsley, or cilantro. For added flavor and to tenderize the meat, you can add fresh lemon or lime juice. Add the marinade and meat, plus a pinch of salt and pepper, to a large sealable plastic bag. Immediately place the bag in the refrigerator and leave it for about 30 minutes. Cook when the 30 minutes is up and don't let it sit in the refrigerator. In addition to marinating, I also recommend baking the meat for a few minutes prior to putting it on the grill. This way, it'll spend less time over high heat while still adding flavor.

# STEAMING

Steaming is a no-nonsense way to prepare healthy meals. Nutrients are retained, and other than water, no additional ingredients are required. To get started, you'll need a steamer. These are often made of either metal (which is often collapsible or a basket that fits in your pot) or bamboo (often double-tiered which is great for steaming multiple types of food at the same time). Start by filling a pot or wok with water and bring to a boil. Toss your food in the steamer and place it over the boiling water, tightly covered. Once the food is vibrantly cooked, remove it from the heat and add flavor by incorporating citrus (orange, lemon, lime), sea salt, freshly ground pepper, or other spices.

I love steaming boneless white chicken breasts (8-10 minutes), shrimp (8-10 minutes), broccoli florets (5-7 minutes), bell peppers (4-6 minutes), baby potatoes (8-12 minutes), carrots (7-10 minutes), kale (4-7 minutes), swiss chard (3-5 minutes), zucchini (5-7 minutes), and green beans (6-10 minutes).

# BLANCHING

This technique is fabulous for making veggies crisp, tender, bright, and easy to store in the freezer. Here's how it's done: Start by boiling water and don't forget to add a pinch or two of salt! Next, prepare an ice bath. Grab a large container and fill it with ice water. Immerse the food into the boiling water for about two to three minutes, then strain and transfer to the ice bath immediately until the food is cooled. Remove it from the water and pat dry. Easy, quick and healthy! Wondering what foods are best for blanching? Try carrot sticks, green beans, broccoli and fennel.

# SAUTÉING

To sauté, you'll need a sauté pan and a little oil. I like to sauté with pure olive oil, organic expeller-pressed canola oil, sesame oil, and occasionally coconut oil. If you're concerned about going too heavy on the oil ('cause there are like, 120 calories in one tablespoon!), you can try an oil sprayer. These often minimize the amount of oil needed.* Let the pan get hot, add your oil, and then add your ingredients. Be sure not to overcrowd the pan and keep the food moving often (toss, flip, and move it around). The word sauté actually comes from the French word sauter, meaning to "flip." The key is to occasionally flip the food and keep the pan hot. Fish fillets, shrimp, beef tenderloin, and thin chicken breasts are great for sautéing. Tender veggies are also a great choice.

*When choosing a spray, avoid ones with petroleum-based propellants and other questionable additives.*

# ROASTING

Roasting uses dry heat and creates meals that are tender, succulent, and full of nutrients. Start by preheating your oven to 400°F. Next, add your meat, vegetables, or fruit to a roasting dish. Dash on your favorite spices and transfer to the oven. You'll want to give veggies and fruit their space, so try not to bunch them all together, and do your best to keep them in a single layer. Set the timer for about 25 minutes. Check your meat temperature to ensure that it's thoroughly cooked and simply keep an eye on the vegetables to be sure they look crisp and not mushy. Once the food is cooked, enjoy it! If it needs a few more minutes, leave it. Which foods are fabulous roasted? Beef, chicken, and fish! You might also enjoy roasted vegetables like potatoes, peppers, broccoli, green beans, Brussels sprouts, carrots, eggplant, parsnips, squash, and zucchini. I also like playing around with roasted fruit like pineapple and whole grapes.

## ADOPT A JUNK-FREE FOOD PHILOSOPHY

We're living in a world where junk food rules and "healthy" food really isn't even that healthy. I get that it's often hard to know what's actually the best food to put into your body. When you're needing to eat low FODMAP to manage your symptoms, it can be hard to see past the challenge of it all or maybe even to care at all how nutrient-rich a food is as long as it's low FODMAP.

And let's just be honest with each other. Frankly, it might be easy to choose low FODMAP junk food just because it won't cause symptoms. But here's my advice: Just because you can chew and swallow it and it's low FODMAP, doesn't necessarily mean that you *should* eat it. Yes, Swedish Fish, Peeps, Dum Dums, Jolly Ranchers, Nerds, Sweet Tarts, Sour Patch Kids, and Smarties are low FODMAP. But remember this: Low FODMAP doesn't mean it's healthy (low FODMAP candy is still just candy). Let's get serious. I seriously think you should steer clear of the processed stuff. Why? Because it's loaded with artificial colors (*Hello, Red Dye #40!*), chemicals, and worst of all, sugar. And I get it that sugar (sucrose/table sugar) is low on the FODMAP scale, but from my years doing this, I've noticed one of the best ways to help individuals feel a better sense of overall well-being is to get them to dramatically decrease their intake of added sugar.

So, because I care about you (*not because I'm trying to drive you crazy*), I don't include white or brown sugar to any of my recipes. And, I recommend low FODMAP products that don't contain any sugar (cane sugar, evaporated cane syrup, brown sugar, sugar in the raw), numbers (blue #2, yellow #5, polysorbate 80), or chemicals (skip anything scary sounding, like monosodium glutamate, azodicarbonamide, and sodium benzoate). I'm trying to get you to eat real food!

Eat *real* low FODMAP foods, feel *real* good

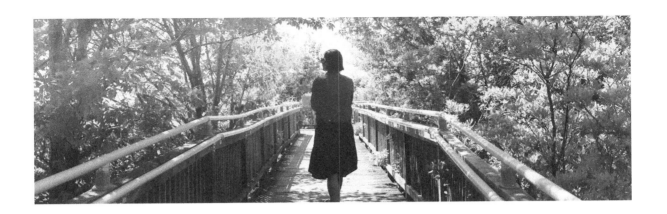

# TOTAL BODY WELLNESS TIPS

Health is so much more than just the absence of disease. It's wellness of mind, body, and spirit. By now *you know* that I feel strongly about food. What you eat matters when it comes to how you feel and how you heal, and while food is often the focus of my health-promoting prescription, there's a lot more to feeling great than just eating great food. I think there are four foundations of health and prevention: Nutrition, physical activity, stress management, and sleep. I could write a few books on each of these topics, but in this book, I want to focus on the most important things you can do right now to feel your best.

## NUTRITION

When it comes to nutrition and weight management, you can eat the healthiest, best foods for your body and be overweight. Yes, you read this right. It can be absolutely maddening if you miss this concept. People ask me all the time if the FODMAP diet is a good weight loss diet. The answer? It depends. It's not that you can't lose weight on the diet (lots of people do!), it's because if you eat too much of any food, you'll gain weight.

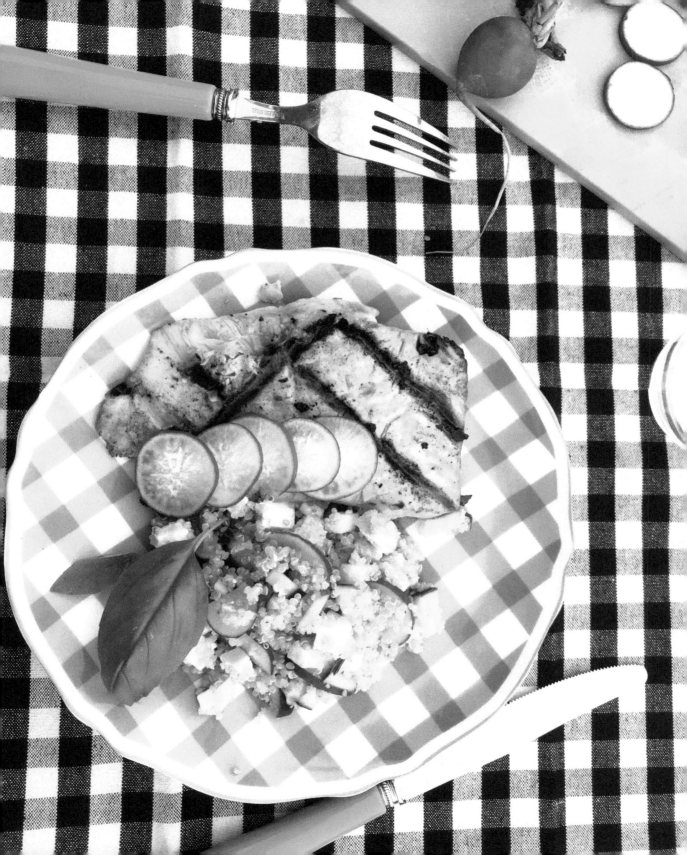

There are 3,500 calories stored in every pound of fat. Meaning, if you consume 500 calories less than your body is burning or burn off 500 calories through exercise each day for seven days, you'll lose a pound of fat in one week. The concept is relatively simple. The execution, however, is a huge challenge for many people.

Let me break this down a little bit further for you. Energy balance is the key to managing a healthy weight. If you take in more calories than your body burns, you'll gain weight. If you take in the same amount of calories that your body burns, you'll stay the same weight. And, if you take in fewer calories than you burn, you'll lose weight. This means you can lose weight eating carrot cake and gain weight eating carrots. I know that sounds crazy, but it's true. You can lose weight eating total junk (just really small portions of it) and gain weight eating super healthy foods (high portions of it or lots of calorie-packed healthy foods like avocado, olive oil, and walnuts). You've got to watch portions and avoid portion distortion!

{**Portion Distortion**: Not knowing how many calories are in the foods you eat and eating too much of it (healthy or junky). Avoid portion distortion by eating small amounts and listening to your body. Pay attention to signals of fullness and be mindful of how much you're consuming.}

Now, just because you *can* eat tasty junk food and maintain a healthy weight doesn't mean you *should*. Let's get real, that's a bad strategy. While energy balance is the key to a healthy weight, the quality of food that you eat determines how you feel, how bloated your belly is, and how your body is able to prevent and fight disease. To achieve your best health through nutrition, you've got to combine two concepts. You've got to eat to your body's metabolism (the right portions of food and amount of calories for your body) while choosing the right kinds of quality, nutrient-dense, low FODMAP, whole foods.

# PHYSICAL ACTIVITY

When it comes to physical activity, movement is key for a healthy body. But, if you've got a sensitive system, you've got to choose the right kinds of exercise. Over-exercise can actually increase digestive symptoms. You've got to get the right kinds of exercise in the right amounts.

Ready for this? Here's an excerpt from a study in the *Journal of Clinical Sports Medicine*: "Exercise can have significant effects on gastrointestinal diseases. Regular, moderate exercise can impart beneficial effects for the intestinal microbiome, irritable bowel syndrome symptoms, and inflammatory bowel disease. High-intensity training or prolonged endurance training, on the other hand, can have negative effects on these same entities. Female athletes report a higher prevalence of irritable bowel syndrome and celiac disease." Too little, not good. Too much, not good. You've got to find just the right amount of exercise for your body *and* you've got to be consistent. I am all about moving your body in a comfortable way, every day.

Another study in the *World Journal of Gastroenterology* showed that regular exercise like walking, cycling, and aerobics has "positive long-term effects on IBS symptoms." Another gut-friendly form of exercise is yoga. The key to success is finding a type of movement you like, one that feels comfortable, and doing it regularly. Not only can exercise help you to manage your gastrointestinal issues, it's shown to decrease depression, blood pressure, risk of cancer, cardiovascular disease, and diabetes. Exercise also improves sleep, muscle tone, and overall quality of life. You've got to just do it.

# STRESS MANAGEMENT

Stress management is another foundation for wellness. How well you manage stress can determine how well your body heals. The good news is that as you begin to manage your digestive symptoms, you'll naturally experience less stress. The less pain, uncertainty and discomfort you face, the less stressed you'll be about social, family, and work-related situations. Less gas, more fun! With that being said, there's more stress than just IBS stress. Life is loaded with it. While you can't often control the stress of life, you can control your body's response to stress.

I am a huge fan of biofeedback. Ever heard of it? It's a way to manage your body's stress reaction by responding to the physiological feedback your body provides. You can either visit a biofeedback practitioner who will hook you up to monitors, show you your body's reactions (signals like muscle tension (EMG), neurological signals (EEG), heart function (EKG), temperature), or you can try DIY methods. Devices like HeartMath, emWave, stress thermometers, and Mindfield GSR sensors can show you how to reap the benefits of biofeedback in the comfort of your home.

Looking for other ways to manage your stress? Try yoga, hiking, meditation, exercise, journaling, cognitive behavioral therapy, time outdoors, hours unplugged, and progressive muscle relaxation. I also highly recommend ditching the doubters, haters, soul suckers, and negative Nancy(s). Social media detoxes are also a great way to eliminate comparison stress without expensive therapy.

# SLEEP

And last but not least, is sleep. You need it, and you probably aren't getting enough of it. One study of 170 on-call doctors with low sleep scores showed a correlation between lack of sleep and onset of functional digestive disorders. In other words, less sleep equals more bowel irritability. You've got to shoot for at least 7½ hours each night. To do this, get yourself in a rhythm. Go to bed at the same time every night and try to wake up the same time every morning, even on the weekends. Ben Franklin's wise words resonate in my head every day: "Early to bed, early to rise makes a (wo)man healthy, wealthy and wise." And while binge watching, social surfing, and night noshing are fun in the moment, they aren't best for you in the long run. Go to bed early, wake up early, feel better.

Here's the bottom line. You've got to build a firm foundation for yourself and your health. To make that foundation strong, focus on the big four: Nutrition, physical activity, stress management, and sleep. Be consistent, and you'll be on your way to the healthiest version of you.

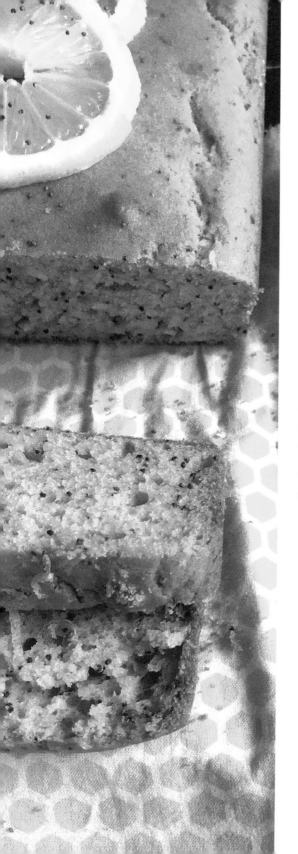

# HAVE YOUR CAKE AND EAT IT TOO

So, cool girl, you are well on your way to making healthy happen! You can have your low FODMAP cake and eat it, too. You now have got all you need to make this low FODMAP style of eating work for your lifestyle. Start with your elimination. Give it a month or two (sometimes even three!) and allow your body to reset. Next, get yourself going with the challenge phase. Work through each of the FODMAP groups and find your triggers. Then, reintroduce the groups you know are safe for you and move on with your life! You'll be feeling cooler, healthier, confident and better. Nothing tastes as good as being healthy and confident feels.

Here's my final thought for you: Remember, more than anything, your mindset matters. If you think you can do this, you will. If you focus on the foods you can have, you won't lament the ones you need to avoid (for now). If you set your mind towards success, you will achieve it.

**Okay, it's up to you now — go get it. Live long, live strong, live #FODMAPfabulous!**

# FODMAP FOOD LIST

## LOWER FODMAP OPTIONS

Low FODMAP foods are safe to consume, but remember that portions matter.
Any food that contains carbohydrates can become a high FODMAP food and
trigger symptoms with increased portions.

### LOW FODMAP FRUIT

Banana - 1 medium (112g)

Blueberries - ¼ cup heaped (40g)

Cantaloupe - ½ cup (90g)

Clementines - 1 medium (86g)

Cumquats - 4 fruits (76g)

Dragon Fruit - 1 medium (330g)

Grapes - 1 cup (150g)

Honeydew - ½ cup (90g)

Kiwi - 2 small peeled (150g)

Lemon - 1 teaspoon (6g)

Lime - 1 teaspoon (6g)

Mandarin Oranges - 2 small (125g)

Orange - 1 medium (130g)

Passionfruit - 1 whole pulp (23g)

Pineapple - 1 cup, chopped (140g)

Raspberries - 10 berries (45g)

Rhubarb - 1 cup, chopped (130g)

Starfruit - 1 medium (94g)

Strawberries - 10 medium (140g)

*Note: Bananas that are overly ripe can become high FODMAP. Choose bananas without brown spots.*

### LOW FODMAP DAIRY

Brie - 2 wedges (40g)

Butter - 1 tablespoon (19g)

Cheddar - 2 slices (40g)

Colby - 2 slices (40g)

Cottage Cheese - 4 tablespoons (36g)

Feta - ½ cup, crumbled) (125g)

Goat Cheese - ½ cup, crumbled (125g)

Goat Milk Yogurt - ½ cup (170g)

Havarti - 1 slices (54g)

Lactose-Free Milk - 1 cup (257g)

Lactose-Free Yogurt - ½ cup (170g)

Mozzarella - ½ cup, grated (60g)

Pecorino and Parmesan - ⅓ cup, grated (40g)

Ricotta - 2 tablespoons (40g)

Swiss - 2 slices (54g)

## LOW FODMAP DAIRY FREE ALTERNATIVES

Almond Milk - 1 cup, 250ml (240g)

Macadamia Milk - 1 cup, 250 ml (240g)

Canned Coconut Milk - ⅓ cup (80g)

Rice Milk - ¾ cup, 200ml (200g)

Hemp Milk - 1 cup, 250ml (240g)

## LOW FODMAP VEGGIES

Alfalfa - ½ cup (17g)

Kale - 1 cup, chopped (137g)

Arugula - 1 cup (35g)

Lettuce - 1 cup (72g)

Bean Sprouts - ½ cup (50g)

Nori - 2 sheets (5g)

Bok Choy - 1 cup (85g)

Olives - 15 small, ½ cup (60g)

Broccoli (Heads) - 1 cup (90g)

Parsnips - ½ cup (62g)

Brussels Sprouts - 2 sprouts (38g)

Potato - 1 medium (122g)

Cabbage (common or red) - 1 cup (94g)

Radish - 2 radish (40g)

Carrot - 1 medium (61g)

Red Peppers - ½ cup (52g)

Collard Greens - 1 cup chopped (36g)

Spaghetti Squash - 1 cup, cooked (155g)

Cucumber - ½ cup (64g)

Spinach - 1 ½ cup (75g)

Eggplant - ½ cup (41g)

Squash - 2 squash (70g)

Fennel - ½ cup (12g)

Swiss Chard - 1 cup, chopped (115g)

Ginger - 1 teaspoon (3g)

Tomato - 1 small (119g)

Green Beans (haricot vert) - 12 beans (86g)

Turnip - 1 cup, diced (65g)

Green Onion Tops - 1 tablespoon (16g)

Zucchini - ⅓ cup (65g)

Green Peppers - ½ cup (52g)

*Note: Green onion tops are low FODMAP while the bulbs are high FODMAP.*

## LOW FODMAP NUTS AND SEEDS

Brazil Nuts - 10 nuts (40g)

Peanuts - 32 nuts (28g)

Chestnuts - 20 nuts (168g)

Pecans - 10 halves (20g)

Chia or Hemp Seeds - 2 tablespoons (24g)

Pine Nuts - 1 tablespoon (14g)

Flaxseeds - 1 tablespoon (15g)

Poppy Seeds - 2 tablespoons (24g)

Macadamia Nuts - 20 nuts (40g)

Pumpkin Seeds - 2 tablespoons (23g)

Sesame Seeds - 1 tablespoon (11g)

Sunflower Seeds - 2 tablespoons, hulled (6g)

Walnuts - 10 nut halves (30g)

*Note: Limit even "safe" nuts to one serving at a time. Even low FODMAP nuts become high FODMAP foods in high quantities.*

# LOW FODMAP PROTEINS

Beef

Chicken

Edamame/soybeans - ½ cup (85g)

Eggs

Fish

Pork Tenderloin

Shrimp

Tofu and Tempeh (firm)

Turkey

*Note: Meats that aren't marinated are always low FODMAP & safe. Make sure that the protein you choose is not marinated with high FODMAP ingredients. You'll be amazed at how many times what you think is "plain" actually includes questionable ingredients.*

# LOW FODMAP GRAINS

Buckwheat Groats - ¾ cup, cooked (135g)

Cornstarch/Flour - ⅔ cup (100g)

Gluten-Free Oats - 1 cup, uncooked (105g)

Gluten-Free Pasta - 1 cup, cooked (145g)

Millet - ⅔ cup (100g)

Polenta - 1 cup, cooked (255g)

Popcorn - 7 cups (120g)

Potato starch - ⅔ cup (100g)

Quinoa - 1 cup, cooked (155g)

Rice - 1 cup, cooked (190g)

Sorghum flour - ⅔ cup (100g)

# LOW FODMAP SWEETENERS

Coconut Sugar - 1 teaspoon (4g)

Palm Sugar - 1 tablespoon (13g)

Pure Maple Syrup - 1 tablespoon (20g)

Rice Malt Syrup - 1 tablespoon (28g)

Stevia - 2 sachets (2g)

*Note: Brown sugar, white sugar, cane syrup, raw sugar, and beet sugar are all low FODMAP, but quite frankly, they're bad for your body. Try to steer clear for better health overall.*

# HIGH FODMAP FOODS

During the elimination phase, you've got to avoid the foods that are high in fermentable carbohydrates. I'm providing you with a list of foods that are high in FODMAPs and the portion size by which they tested as high. You can reset your digestive system and get relief when you keep your FODMAP load low.

*Fewer Fermentable Carbs = Fewer Symptoms*

## HIGH FODMAP FRUIT

Apple - 1 medium (165g)

Apricot - 2 apricots (112g)

Avocado - ½ whole avocado (80g)

Blackberries - 10 berries (50g)

Cherries - 6 cherries (42g)

Dried currants - 2 tablespoons (26g)

Figs - 4 figs (76g)

Grapefruit - 1 medium (207g)

Guava - (unripe) ½ medium (117g)

Lychee - 10 (104g)

Mango - 1 mango (207g)

Nectarine - 1 medium (151g)

Peach - 1 medium (145g)

Pear - 1 medium (166g)

Plum - 1 plum (66g)

Pomegranate - ½ cup seeds (76g)

Raisins - 2 tablespoons (26g)

Watermelon - 1 thick slice (286g)

## HIGH FODMAP DAIRY

Cow Milk - 1 cup, 250 ml (257g)

Cream Cheese - 4 tablespoons (81g)

Goat Milk - 1 cup, 250 ml (257g)

Ice Cream - 2 level scoops (88g)

Kefir - 200 ml (200g)

Ricotta - 4 tablespoons (80g)

Sheep Milk - 1 cup, 250 ml (257g)

Sour Cream - ½ cup, 125ml (126g)

## HIGH FODMAP VEGGIES

Artichokes - ½ small globe (50g)

Asparagus - 2 spears (30g)

Beetroot - 4 slices (41g)

Broccoli Stalks - 1 cup (90g)

Butternut Squash - ½ cup, diced (60g)

Cabbage (savoy) - 1 cup (70g)

Cauliflower - ½ cup (66g)

Celery - ½ medium stalk/12cm (19g)

Corn - 1 cob (85g)

Garlic - 1 clove (3g)

Green Onion Bulb - 2 teaspoons (8g)

Leek - 1 leek (83g)

Mushroom - 1 mushroom (84g)

Onion - ½ onion (45g)

Peas - ½ cup (72g)

Pumpkin - ½ cup, diced (60g)

Shallot - 1 shallot (6g)

Snow Peas - 10 pods (33g)

Sugar Snap Peas - ½ cup (60g)

Sun-Dried Tomato - 4 pieces (16g)

Sweet Potato - 1 cup (140g)

Taro - 1 cup, diced (164g)

## HIGH FODMAP NUTS

Almonds - 20 nuts (24g)

Cashews - 20 nuts (30g)

Hazelnuts - 20 nuts (30g)

Pistachio - 30 nuts (23g)

## HIGH FODMAP LEGUMES

Beans (except green beans) - ¼ cup (45g) to ½ cup (91g)

Chickpeas (sprouted) - ½ cup (84g)

Hummus - 2 tablespoons (40g)

Lentils - ½ cup (46g)

## HIGH FODMAP SWEETENERS

Agave - 1 tablespoon (21g)

High Fructose Corn Syrup

Honey - 2 tablespoons (56g)

Molasses Syrup - ½ tablespoon

Sugar Alcohols: Xylitol, Isomalt, Mannitol, Maltitol, Sorbitol

## HIGH FODMAP GRAINS

Barley - 1 cup, cooked (225g)

Chickpea Flour - ⅔ cup (95g)

Coconut Flour - ⅔ cup (100g)

Kamut - ⅔ cup (100g)

Rye - ⅔ cup (95g)

Spelt - ⅔ cup (100g)

Wheat - ⅔ cup (100g)

*Note: Avoid anything containing gluten. Though gluten itself is not a high FODMAP substance, the foods that contain gluten (wheat, barley, rye) are all high FODMAP.*

# YOU'LL ALSO WANT TO TAKE NOTE OF THESE

Some foods don't naturally fall into a category. So, I put them here.

## OTHER LOW FODMAP INGREDIENTS

Almond Butter

Apple Cider Vinegar

Asafoetida Powder

Capers

Cocoa Powder

Coconut Yogurt

Dried Shredded Coconut

Garlic-Infused Oils

Herbs (Basil, bay leaves, cilantro, cloves, coriander, lemongrass, parsley, rosemary, tarragon, thyme)

Mustard

Oils (Avocado, canola, coconut, olive, peanut, rice bran, sesame, sunflower, vegetables)

Peanut Butter

Pea Protein Powder

Rice Wine Vinegar

Soy Sauce - 2 tablespoons (42g)

Spices (Allspice, cardamom, cinnamon, chili powder, paprika, saffron, turmeric)

Vanilla

Wheatgrass Powder

## OTHER HIGH FODMAP INGREDIENTS

Chicory

Fruit Juice Sweetened Foods

Inulin

Ketchup

Onion/Garlic Powder

Pesto (When made with garlic and onions)

Tahini (When made with garlic)

## WHAT TO DRINK

Water, weakly brewed unsweetened black, white or green tea (hot or cold), peppermint tea, black coffee

## WHAT NOT TO DRINK

Alcohol, coconut water, lattes, juice, chai tea, chamomile tea, fennel tea, herbal tea, oolong tea, beverages containing high-fructose corn syrup

*Note: There are certain types of alcohol, like gin, whiskey, and red wine that are considered low FODMAP. However, for overall health reasons, I strongly recommend not drinking beverages containing alcohol.*

# THE FODMAP DIET: IT'S A SCIENCE AND AN ART

It's really about making FODMAPs work for you. As more research is being done, the quantities of all different types of foods are being tested and retested at varying portions to determine their fermentability and how they could potentially affect a sensitive individual.

It's why on some lists you'll see a food categorized as low FODMAP and on others you'll see that same food listed as moderate or high. It really depends on the portion size the author is taking into consideration. Take zucchini for example: If you eat 1/3 cup or less, you're in the safe zone. More than 1/3 cup and that same zucchini might cause symptoms you if you're sensitive to oligos. I've also seen honeydew melon listed some places as low FODMAP and other places as high FODMAP. Why? Because 1/2 cup of honeydew is shown to be low FODMAP whereas 1 cup tests high. Test yourself and listen to your body. Use the research as a guide and make it work for you!

---

## YOU CAN DO IT!

The Bentson kitchen has been extra busy these days — To ensure that each recipe in this book is easy to make and tastes great, my super cool boys, Ben (8 years old) and Grey (4 years old), have tested each recipe. If they can do it, you can do it too!

*-dr KB*

---

# LOW FODMAP RECIPES

## BREAKFAST

01. Easy Banana French Toast
[N, D, P]

02. Create Your Own Frittata
[N, D, P]

03. Oh-So-Good Oatmeal
[N, D, P, V, E]

04. Morning Glory Smoothie
[N, D, P, V, E]

05. Blueberry Maple Muffins
[N, D, P, V, E]

06. Crepes Sweet or Savory
[N, D, P]

07. Good Quiche
[N, P]

08. Blueberry Fritters
[N, D, P]

09. Orange Pecan Granola
[D, P, V, E]

10. Yogurt Parfait

## LUNCH/DINNER

11. Stir Fried Shrimp and Rice Noodles
[N, D, P]

12. Soy, Sesame Maple Salmon
[N, D, P, E]

13. Kale, Orange & Feta Salad with Citrus Dressing
[N, P]

14. Chicken Pecan Grape Salad Sandwich
[D, P]

15. Rotini Pasta with Cherry Tomato and Arugula
[N, P]

16. Chicken Fried Rice
[N, D, P]

17. Chicken and Wild Rice Soup
[N, D, P, E]

18. Pan-Seared Steak
[N, D, P, E]

19. Turkey Tacos
[N, D, P, E]

20. Veggie Noodles with Pesto and Cherry Tomato
[D, P]

21. Lemon Chicken
[N, D, P]

22. Niçoise Salad with Tuna
[N, D, P]

23. Roasted Red Peppers with Tomato Sauce and Pasta
[N, D, P, V, E]

24. Stuffed Peppers
[N, P, E]

25. Wild Rice, Zucchini, Fennel and Walnuts
[D, P, V, E]

26. Beef and Broccoli
[N, D, P, E]

27. Gazpacho
[N, D, P]

28. Simple Bacon and Egg Salad
[N, D, P]

29. Tomato Basil Millet
[N, D, P, V, E]

30. Broccoli and Bacon Salad
[N, D, P]

## ON THE SIDE

## TREATS

## ALLERGY GUIDE FOR FODMAP RECIPES

N = Tree Nut Free

P = Peanut Free

D = Dairy Free

V = Vegan

E = Egg Free

*NOTE: ALL recipes are gluten-free and contain no refined sugar*

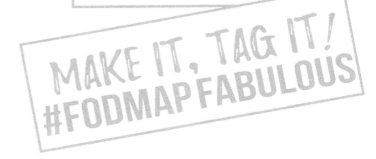

MAKE IT, TAG IT!
#FODMAPFABULOUS

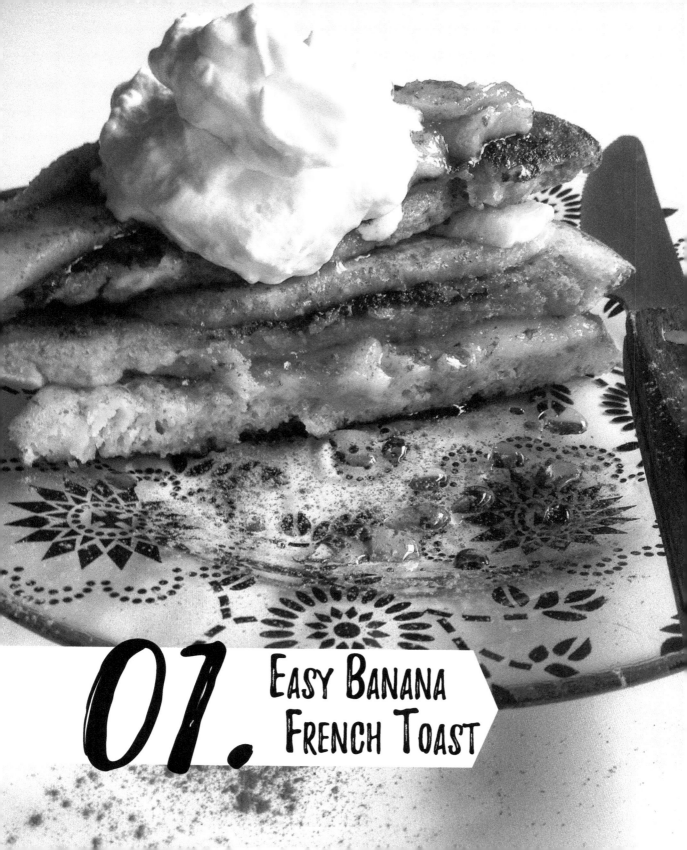

# 07. Easy Banana French Toast

# EASY BANANA FRENCH TOAST
MAKES 4-6 SLICES OF FRENCH TOAST

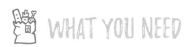 WHAT YOU NEED

## FRENCH TOAST

2 bananas

3 beaten eggs

⅛ teaspoon cinnamon

⅛ teaspoon ginger

⅛ teaspoon nutmeg

½ teaspoon vanilla extract

4-6 slices gluten free bread

2-3 tablespoons coconut oil

## COCONUT WHIPPED CREAM (optional)

1 can full-fat refrigerated coconut milk

1 tablespoon pure maple syrup

## TOPPINGS

Sliced banana

Pure maple syrup

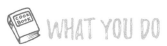 WHAT YOU DO

## PREPARE THE FRENCH TOAST

1. Using a potato masher or a fork, mash the banana. Then, in a shallow mixing bowl, whisk the mashed banana with the beaten egg, cinnamon, ginger, nutmeg, and vanilla to make the batter.

2. Dip the bread into the batter. Allow each slice of bread to fully absorb the mix.

3. Add ½ tablespoon of coconut oil to a flat pan or large sauté pan on medium heat. Once melted, add the battered bread slices. Add additional ½ tablespoon as needed to keep the pan oiled.

4. Cook each slice on medium heat until golden brown. You'll likely cook each side for about two to three minutes. Use a thin spatula to flip the toast at about two minutes (or until golden brown).

## PREPARE THE FRESH WHIPPED CREAM

1. In a large mixing bowl, add cold (this is very important) full-fat coconut milk and maple syrup. Use a mixer at high speed to create the cream. Mix until gentle peaks form.

2. Serve the French toast hot and topped with a touch of fresh whipped cream, a few banana slices, and pure maple syrup.

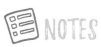 NOTES

✓ Look for gluten-free bread that doesn't have honey, high fructose corn syrup, or inulin and isn't fruit juice sweetened with high FODMAP fruit like pear or apple.

✓ If you don't have celiac disease, you may be able to tolerate fresh sourdough bread.

✓ Use organic eggs to avoid added hormones, antibiotics, pesticides, and GMOs.

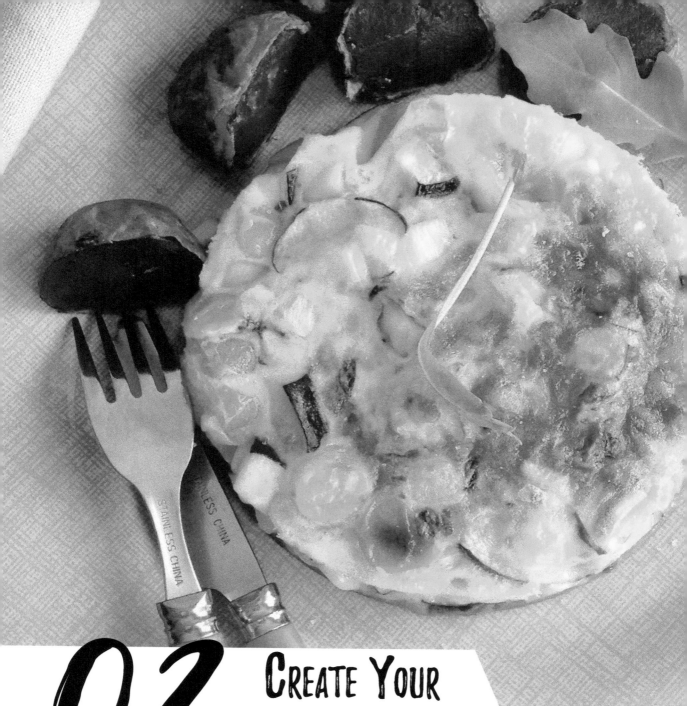

# 02. Create Your Own Frittata

# CREATE YOUR OWN FRITTATA
SERVES 4-6

 WHAT YOU NEED

6-8 extra large eggs

1-2 teaspoons fresh or dried herbs (oregano, thyme, basil, rosemary)

Olive oil

1 teaspoon salt

½ teaspoon freshly ground pepper

**FILLING: CHOOSE THREE OR FOUR FAVORITES**

½ cup diced tomatoes

½ cup diced zucchini

¼ cup baby arugula

1 medium potato, diced

1 medium red bell pepper, diced

½ cup broccoli florets, heads

 WHAT YOU DO

1. Start by preheating the oven to 400-450°F.

2. Heat 1-2 teaspoons of oil in a 10- to 12-inch nonstick frying pan or cast iron skillet until oil is warm. You can test this with the palm of your hand 2-3 inches above the pan. Choose three or four of your favorite low fodmap vegetables. Add the slower cooking vegetables (like broccoli and potato) to the pan first. Once slightly tender, add the remaining vegetables and cook thoroughly. Season with ½ teaspoon salt, ¼ teaspoon pepper, and 1 teaspoon of herbs. Use a spatula to evenly distribute the vegetables over the bottom of the pan.

3. In a small mixing bowl, use a whisk to scramble the eggs. Sprinkle in the remaining salt, pepper and herbs.

4. Pour the egg mix over the vegetables making sure that the eggs settle evenly, tilting the pan if necessary. Cook the eggs and vegetables for about one to two minutes until you see the eggs at the edges of the pan starting to set.

5. Once you notice that the eggs are setting at the bottom and sides of the pan, remove the pan from the stove top and place it in the preheated oven. As an alternative, you may also turn on the broiler. Leave the frittata in the oven for about eight to ten minutes, checking frequently. Remove the pan from the heat when the top of the eggs begin to turn golden brown. Cut a small slit into the center to ensure the eggs have fully set. Reminder: The pan will be hot! Don't forget to use an oven mitt.

6. Let the frittata continue to set outside the oven for about three to four minutes. Cut into slices and serve warm.

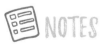 NOTES

✓ The pictured filling is tomato, zucchini, and arugula.

✓ Use organic eggs to avoid added hormones, antibiotics, pesticides, and GMOs.

LOOKING FOR PERFECT POTATOES? LOOK NO FURTHER THAN RECIPE #31.

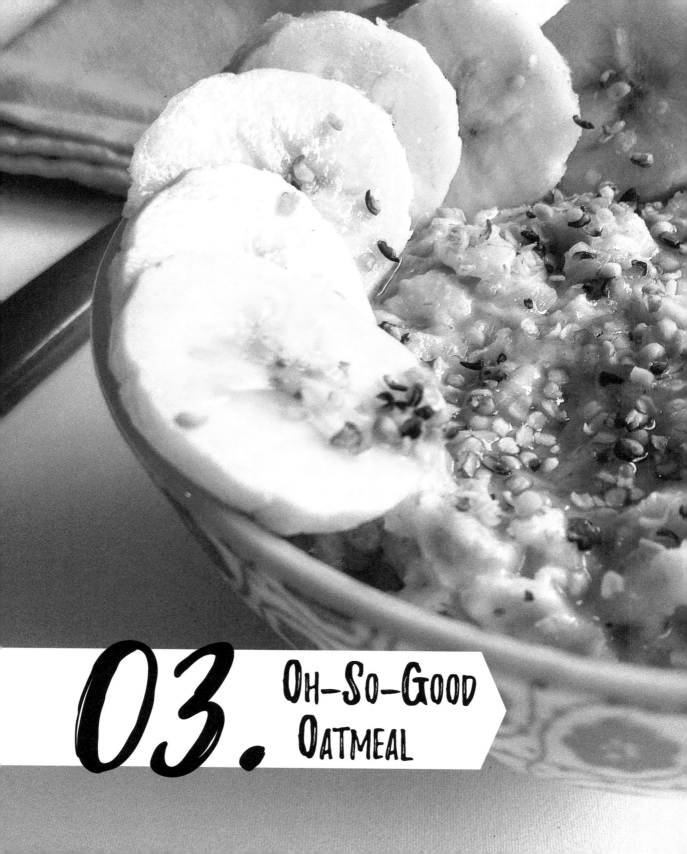

# 03. Oh-So-Good Oatmeal

# Oh-So-Good Oatmeal
SERVES 4-6

 WHAT YOU NEED

2 cups water
1 cup quick cooking gluten-free oats
½-1 cup almond milk
Dash vanilla extract

1 large banana
1 tablespoon pure maple syrup
1 tablespoon hemp seeds

 WHAT YOU DO

1. In a medium saucepan, bring two cups of water to a boil.
2. Once boiling, add in the 1 cup of quick-cooking gluten-free oats and reduce the heat to low. Cook the oats for about two to five minutes. Stir frequently.
3. Remove the saucepan from the heat and cover. Let sit for two to three minutes.
4. Using a small saucepan, heat the almond milk and a dash of vanilla extract.
5. Serve cooked oats with warm almond milk and top with sliced banana, maple syrup, and hemp seeds.

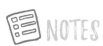 NOTES

✓ To add more flavor, toast hemp seeds by heating them in a small dry skillet until lightly browned.
✓ If you want an alternative to hemp seeds, try chia seeds or ground flax.
✓ For precise measurement, a dash is equal to ⅛ teaspoon.
✓ Don't like bananas? You can substitute with blueberries, raspberries, kiwi, star fruit or strawberries instead.

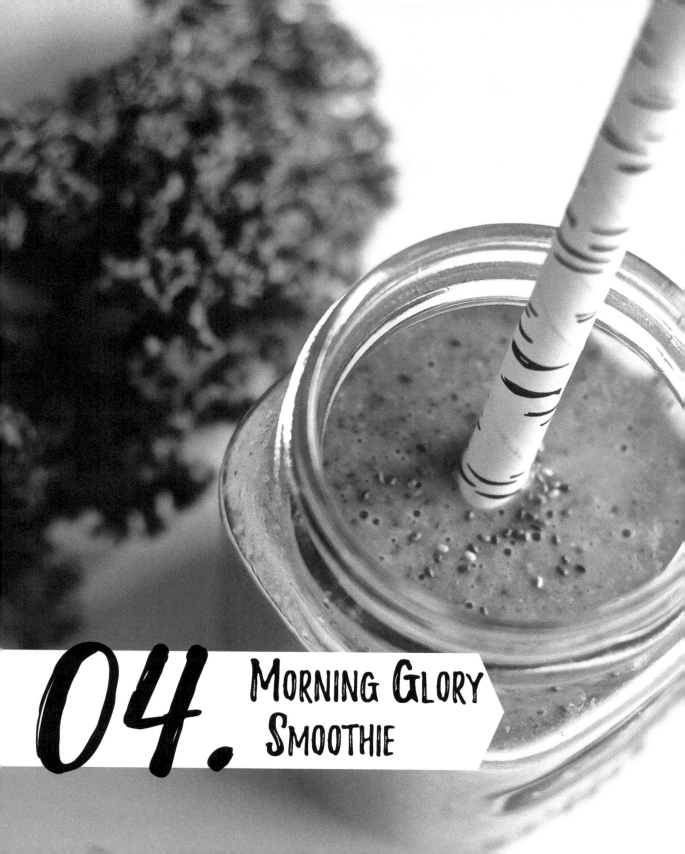

# 04. MORNING GLORY SMOOTHIE

# MORNING GLORY SMOOTHIE
SERVES 4

 WHAT YOU NEED

2 cups water, rice, macadamia, or almond milk

1 cup frozen pineapple chunks

2 bananas

½ cup frozen green grapes

2 cups kale

1 teaspoon chia seeds

 WHAT YOU DO

1. Place all ingredients in the blender and blend until smooth.

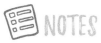 NOTES

✓ Fruit substitutions: Frozen kiwi or honeydew

✓ Green substitutions: Spinach or butter lettuce

✓ Chia seeds substitutions: Hemp hearts, pea protein powder, ground flax

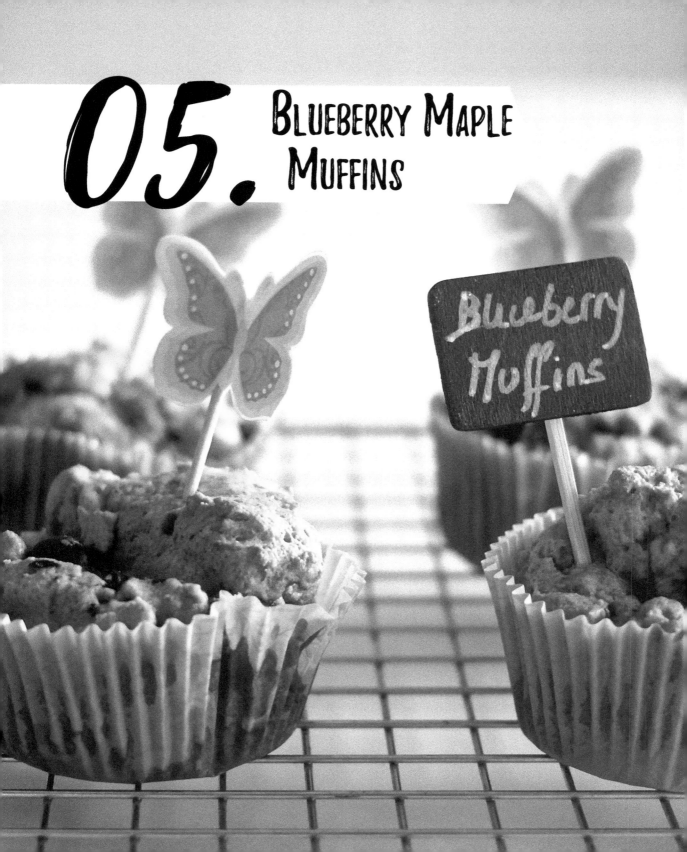

# 05. BLUEBERRY MAPLE MUFFINS

Blueberry Muffins

# BLUEBERRY MAPLE MUFFINS
MAKES 12 MUFFINS

 WHAT YOU NEED

2¼ cups of gluten-free flour*

2 teaspoons baking powder

1 teaspoon baking soda

1 teaspoon salt

⅔ cup pure maple syrup

½ cup coconut oil melted or liquid

⅔ cup almond, rice, or macadamia milk

2 teaspoons pure vanilla extract

⅔ cup fresh blueberries

 WHAT YOU DO

1. Preheat your oven to 325°F.

2. Whisk together gluten-free flour, baking powder, baking soda, and salt in a medium- sized bowl. Next, add in the coconut oil, maple syrup, milk, and vanilla. Stir the ingredients together until the batter becomes smooth.

3. Carefully fold the blueberries into the mixture until they are distributed evenly throughout.

4. Line a 12-cup muffin tin with paper liners. Evenly add the batter to each tin, almost filling them. Bake the muffins for about 20-24 minutes until a toothpick or thin knife can be removed from the center of the muffin without any residue.

5. Once you take the muffins out of the oven, let them rest in the tin for about 12-15 minutes.

6. Transfer muffins to a wire rack to complete the cool-down process. Store in an airtight container (up to three days) or freeze.

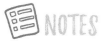 NOTES

✓ *I recommend using all-purpose, gluten-free baking flour. If you use a brand that doesn't contain a binder (like xanthan gum) to replace the gluten, chia seeds or xanthan gum are needed.

✓ Add ¾ teaspoons xanthan gum per 1 cup gluten-free flour. For this recipe, you'll need to add approximately 1½ teaspoons of xanthan gum.

✓ To use chia seeds, substitute one part chia to two parts boiling water. Stir frequently, then let rest for at least five minutes until thickened. Cool to room temperature. For this recipe, you'll need approximately 1½ teaspoons of the chia/water mix (½ teaspoon of chia + 1 teaspoon water).

✓ Don't have fresh blueberries? You can use frozen instead.

✓ Don't have coconut oil? You can use expeller-pressed, organic canola oil instead.

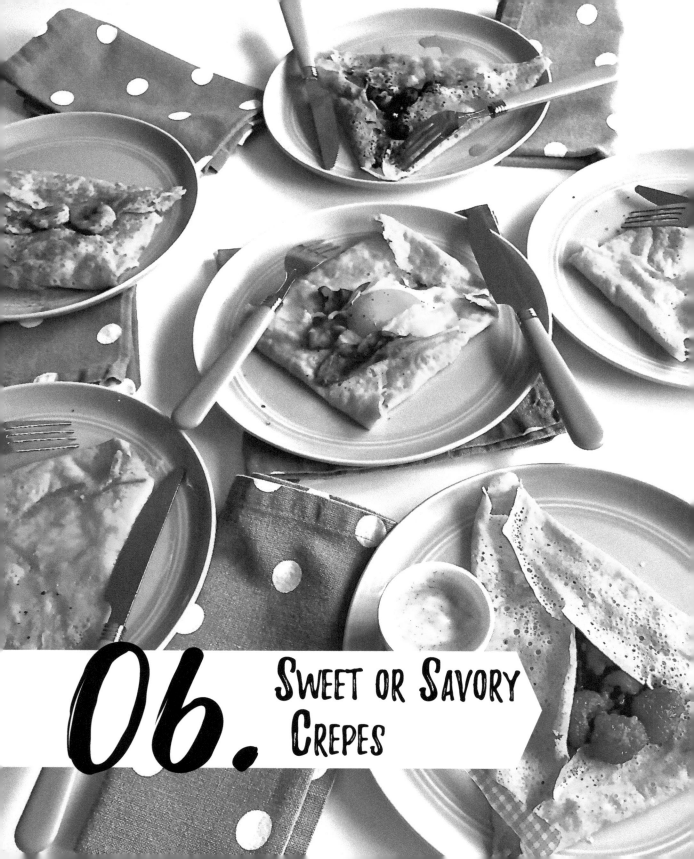

# 06.
## Sweet or Savory Crepes

# SWEET OR SAVORY CREPES *(RECIPE BY PAULINE BONNET DE KERDREL)*

MAKES 8

## WHAT YOU NEED

1 tablespoon coconut oil

2 eggs

2 cups plant-based milk

1 cup gluten-free flour*

Pinch salt

1 tablespoon pure maple syrup or 1 teaspoon coconut sugar

## WHAT YOU DO

1. Coconut oil is a solid at room temperature. For this recipe, you need to liquify the coconut oil. Use a small saucepan over low heat to heat the oil, stirring frequently until it's a liquid.

2. In a small mixing bowl, beat eggs with a whisk.

3. In a large mixing bowl, combine all ingredients by stirring (or beat on low speed with a hand mixer).

4. Allow the mix to rest for about 20-30 minutes at room temperature. If you plan to make the batter ahead of time, it can be covered and stored in the fridge overnight. After refrigeration, mix the batter again by hand or with a mixer.

5. Lightly coat a medium-sized non-stick pan with coconut oil and heat the pan over medium-low heat. Once the pan is hot (test this with the palm of your hand 2-3 inches above the pan), take ⅓ to ½ cup of batter and pour it in the center of the pan until a circle forms. Heat the batter for one to two minutes or until you notice small air bubbles forming in the center and a light brown color around the edges. Flip the crepe with a thin spatula to heat the other side (about one minute) and transfer your crepe to a plate.

6. Choose your favorite sweet or savory fillings and place them in the center of your crepe. Then, fold the crepe from both sides and serve warm.

## Mix-and-Match Crepe Filling

| Sweet | | Savory | |
|---|---|---|---|
| Blueberries | Orange | Steak | Chicken |
| Raspberries | Peanut Butter | Egg | Turkey |
| Kiwi | Coconut Whipped Cream | Spinach | Bacon |
| Strawberries | Maple Syrup | Basil | Swiss Cheese |
| Cinnamon | Lactose-Free Yogurt | | Cheddar Cheese |
| Bananas | Maple Sugar | | |

## NOTES

✓ Safe plant-based milks include: Unsweetened rice (vanilla rice milk gives a sweet crepe great flavor), hemp, macadamia, almond, and quinoa. Not dairy intolerant? You can also use lactose-free milk.

✓ *If you don't use a brand of gluten-free flour that contains a binder to replace the gluten, you need to add xanthan gum.

✓ Add ¾ teaspoons xanthan gum per one cup of gluten-free flour. For this recipe, you'll need to add approximately ¾ teaspoons of xanthan gum.

✓ Use organic eggs to avoid added hormones, antibiotics, pesticides, and GMOs.

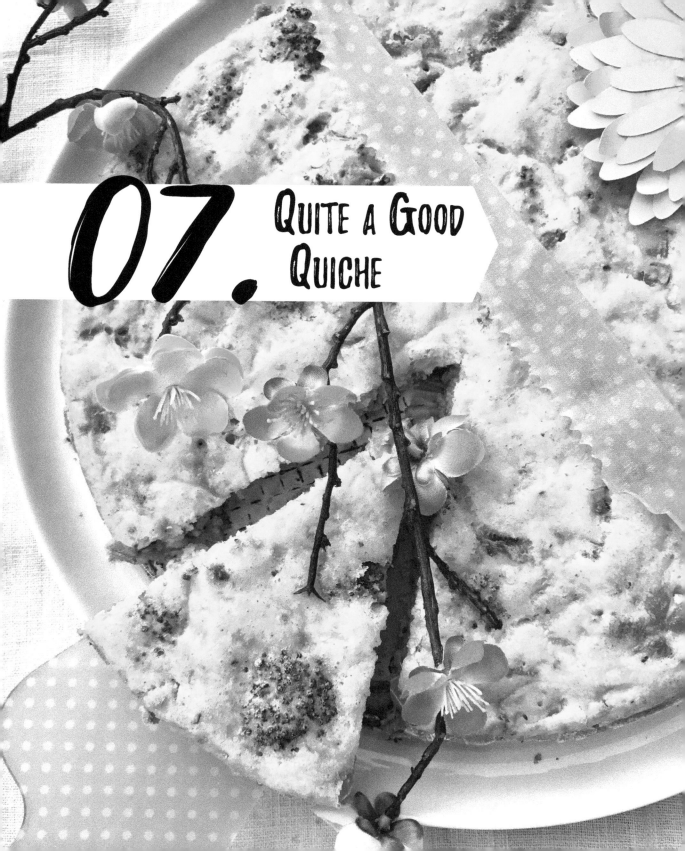

# 07.
## Quite a Good
## Quiche

# QUITE A GOOD QUICHE
SERVES 4

 WHAT YOU NEED

Olive oil

6 eggs

1 cup all-purpose gluten-free flour

1 cup lactose-free milk, unsweetened plain rice, or almond milk

1 cup shredded cheddar, mozzarella, or Swiss

⅓ cup chopped broccoli

⅓ cup chopped tomatoes

4 tablespoons cooked bacon (optional)

Handful of fresh chopped basil (optional)

Pinch salt and fresh-ground pepper

 WHAT YOU DO

1. Start by preheating your oven to 350°F. Grease a pie or quiche dish with olive oil.

2. In a large mixing bowl, beat the eggs with a whisk. Beat in the flour* and milk (or milk alternative). Season with salt and pepper.

3. Gently stir in the cheese, broccoli, and tomatoes (add bacon and basil if desired). Lightly season again with salt.

4. Transfer the mix into the greased dish.

5. Bake uncovered for about 45-50 minutes or until the center is set. You'll know that it's set when you move the dish and the center doesn't jiggle. Let it cool in the dish for about five to seven minutes before serving.

 NOTES

✓ Use organic eggs to avoid added hormones, antibiotics, pesticides, and GMOs.

✓ *If you don't use a brand of gluten-free flour that contains a binder to replace the gluten, you need to add xanthan gum.

✓ Add ¾ teaspoons xanthan gum per one cup gluten-free flour. For this recipe, you'll need to add approximately ¾ teaspoons of xanthan gum.

✓ Look for bacon that's free from nitrates and nitrites, chemicals, onion or garlic powder and added sugar.

✓ Can't tolerate dairy? Substitute the cheddar cheese with soy cheese instead. Up to 40 grams is low FODMAP.

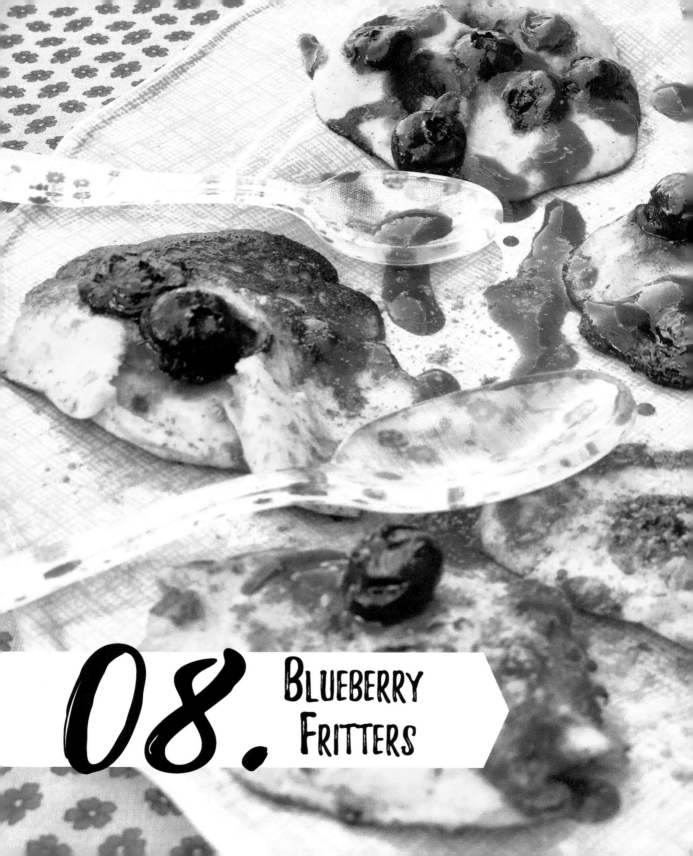

# 08. Blueberry Fritters

# BLUEBERRY FRITTERS
SERVES 4

 WHAT YOU NEED

1 banana

2 eggs, beaten

Pinch of cinnamon

½ teaspoon vanilla

½ teaspoon pure maple syrup

¼-½ cup blueberries

1-2 tablespoons coconut oil

 WHAT YOU DO

1. In a large bowl, use a potato masher to mash the banana. Once the banana is mashed, mix in the beaten egg, cinnamon, vanilla, and maple syrup.

2. Gently stir in blueberries.

3. Heat a large rimmed frying pan over medium heat. Add a little coconut oil to the pan, then place spoonfuls of batter on to it. Allow the batter to cook for about two to four minutes (until edges appear cooked and the batter can be easily moved), then use a thin spatula to flip them over. Heat the other side for about two minutes or until golden brown. Sometimes these are hard to flip — if so, just heat the batter a bit longer until it's cooked through. Serve hot.

 NOTES

✓ These taste delicious with an extra drizzle of maple syrup at the finish.

✓ Using wild blueberries can increase both the flavor and the nutrients.

✓ Fresh blueberries out of season? Try frozen instead.

✓ Use organic eggs to avoid added hormones, antibiotics, pesticides, and GMOs.

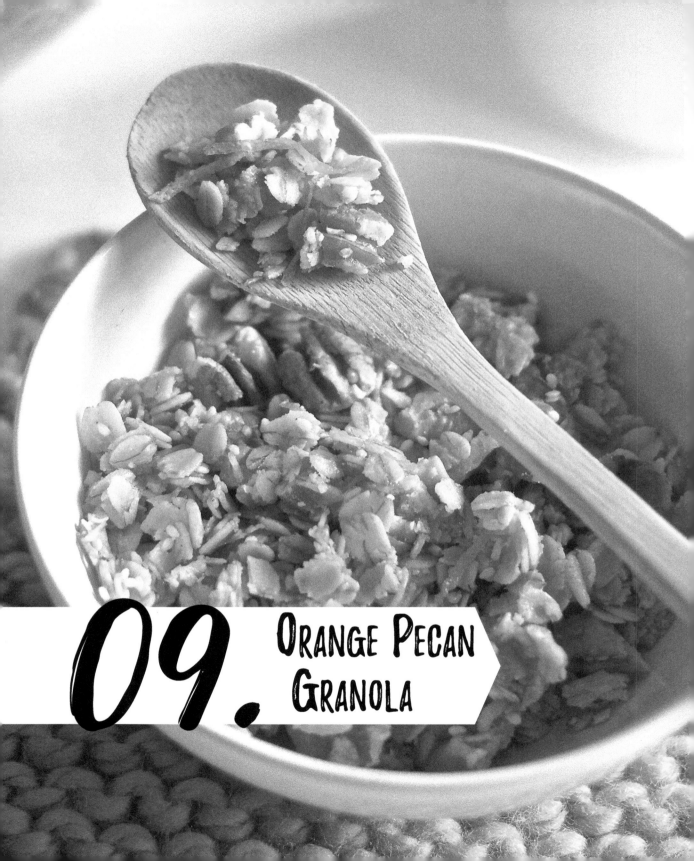

**09.** Orange Pecan Granola

# ORANGE PECAN GRANOLA
SERVES 8-10

 WHAT YOU NEED

½ cup coconut oil

½ cup pure maple syrup

1 teaspoon vanilla extract

3½ cups gluten-free rolled or quick-cooking oats

1½ cups chopped pecans

¼ cup hulled pumpkin or sunflower seeds

1 teaspoon sesame seeds (optional)

Zest of one orange

Pinch of salt

 WHAT YOU DO

1. Preheat the oven to 300°F.
2. In a medium sized mixing bowl, whisk together coconut oil (in liquid form), maple syrup, and vanilla extract.
3. In a large bowl, combine the oats, pecans, seeds, orange zest, and sea salt.
4. Add the wet mixture to the dry. Combine all ingredients by stirring well with a wooden spoon.
5. Line a baking sheet and add the granola mix. Spread the ingredients evenly across the baking sheet.
6. Bake for about 25-28 minutes until golden. Stir the mixture about halfway through baking (13-15 minutes).
7. Remove from heat, but leave on the baking sheet until cool. The granola will crisp as it cools.

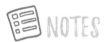 NOTES

✓ Coconut oil is in a solid form at room temperature. To liquify it, simply place it in a saucepan over low heat.

✓ Granola can be stored for up to two weeks in an airtight container.

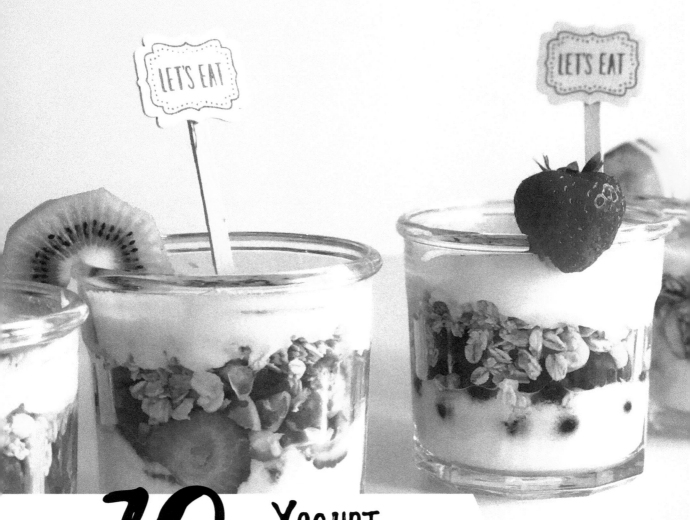

# 10. Yogurt Parfait

# Yogurt Parfait
Makes 4

 ## WHAT YOU NEED

3 cups lactose-free or coconut yogurt

Choose 1 cup of: Blueberries, strawberries, sliced or diced bananas, orange slices, diced kiwi, or pineapple

Choose ½ cup of nuts or seeds: Pumpkins seeds, peanuts, macadamia nuts, pecans, brazil nuts, pine nuts, walnuts, or sesame seeds

Choose 1 cup of cereal or grain: Orange pecan granola (see recipe #9), puffed rice, cooked quinoa, cooked brown rice, or cooked buckwheat

Optional: Drizzle of pure maple syrup, sprinkle of chia seeds, sprinkle of ground flax seeds

 ## WHAT YOU DO

1. Start by adding ⅓ cup of lactose-free yogurt to the bottom of 4 jars or glasses.
2. Next, add a few tablespoons of fruit, nuts/seeds and cereal/grain to the top of your yogurt.
3. Alternate layers of yogurt followed by fruit, nuts and cereal until you reach the top of your jar or glass.
4. Serve immediately.

 ## NOTES

✓ This recipe can be doubled (or tripled!) and makes for the perfect party treat (especially fun when served create-your-own style).

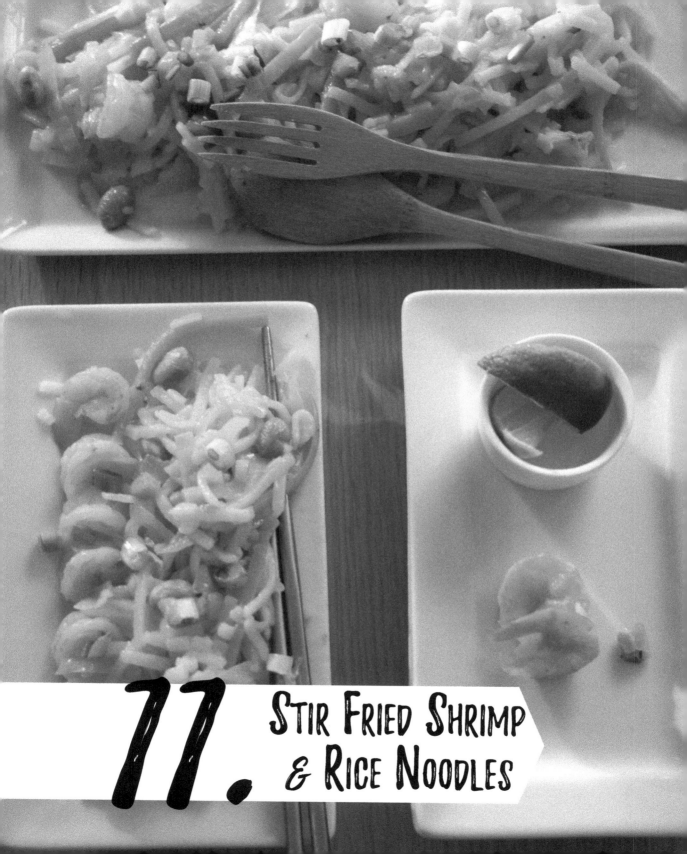

# 11. Stir Fried Shrimp & Rice Noodles

# STIR FRIED SHRIMP AND RICE NOODLES
SERVES 4

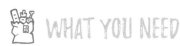 WHAT YOU NEED

## SHRIMP AND RICE NOODLES

1 tablespoon garlic-infused oil (Recipe #39)

1 ½ teaspoon minced ginger

1 pound shrimp, peeled and deveined

2 tablespoon sesame oil

2 large carrots, thickly grated

½ cup cabbage (not savoy), coarsely chopped

¼ cup edamame

8 ounces rice noodles

3 tablespoons soy sauce

3 cups water

## TOPPINGS

Juice of ½ fresh lime

Green onion tops (optional)

 WHAT YOU DO

1. In a large skillet or frying pan, heat the garlic infused oil and minced ginger until warm (test this with the palm of your hand 2-3 inches above the pan). Cook the shrimp for about 5 minutes (stirring frequently) until they're no longer translucent. Remove from the skillet and set aside.

2. In the same skillet or pan, heat the sesame oil. Add the carrots, cabbage, and edamame. Cook until tender (about three to five minutes). Remove from skillet and set aside.

3. In a large pot, bring the water or stock and soy sauce to a boil. Add the noodles and cook until tender. Stir in the cooked vegetables and shrimp.

4. Heat the last tablespoon of sesame oil in the skillet. Add the ingredients from the pot. Stir-fry for about 10 minutes (most of the liquid should be absorbed).

5. Squeeze on the fresh lime. Top with the green onions. Serve warm.

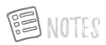 NOTES

✓ The bulbs of green onions are high fodmap, so use only the tops.

✓ Don't prefer or tolerate garlic-infused oil? Use pure olive oil instead.

✓ Use thick or thin rice noodles depending on your preference.

✓ While white rice noodles are fine to use, brown rice noodles are the most nutrient dense option.

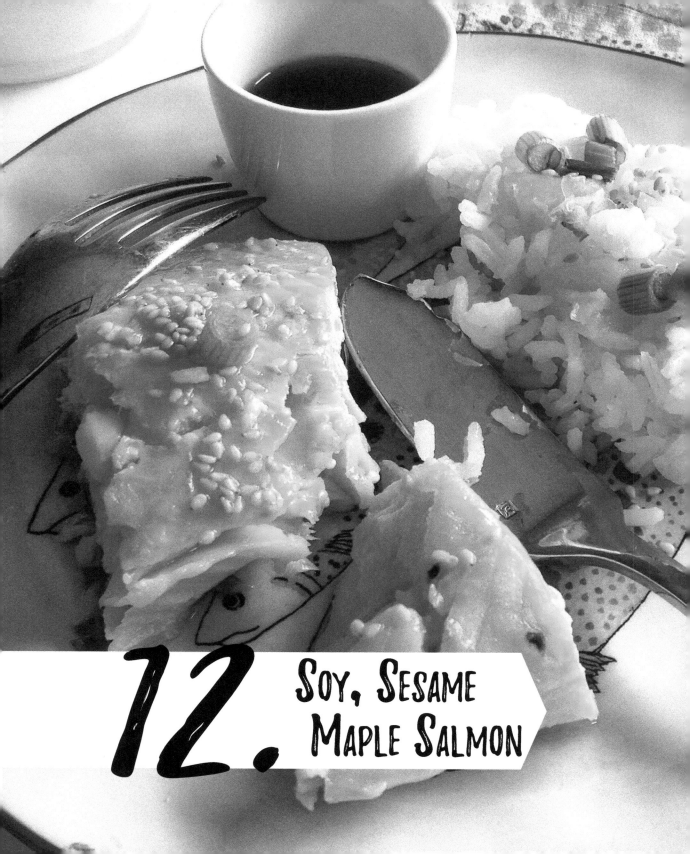

# 12. Soy, Sesame Maple Salmon

# Soy, Sesame Maple Salmon

SERVES 2

 ## WHAT YOU NEED

2 center cut salmon fillets, 6 oz. each

⅓ cup pure maple syrup

2 tablespoons sesame oil

3 tablespoons gluten-free soy sauce

1-2 teaspoons toasted sesame seeds

 ## WHAT YOU DO

1. Start by preheating the oven to 400°F.
2. Whisk together the pure maple syrup and sesame oil. Place the salmon in the marinade and refrigerate for 15-30 minutes (turning once).
3. Line a baking sheet with foil and place the salmon in the center of the sheet. Bake for 15 minutes or until a fork can easily remove flakes from the surface.

**Optional Step:** Make a Glaze. In a saucepan, take the leftover marinade and bring it to a boil. Once boiling, lower the heat and allow to simmer. Drizzle glaze over fully cooked salmon and top with toasted sesame seeds.

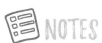 ## NOTES

✓ Salmon can also be grilled, poached or broiled.

✓ Read soy sauce labels carefully and avoid high-fructose corn syrup.

LOOKING FOR PINEAPPLE RICE? LOOK NO FURTHER THAN RECIPE #32.

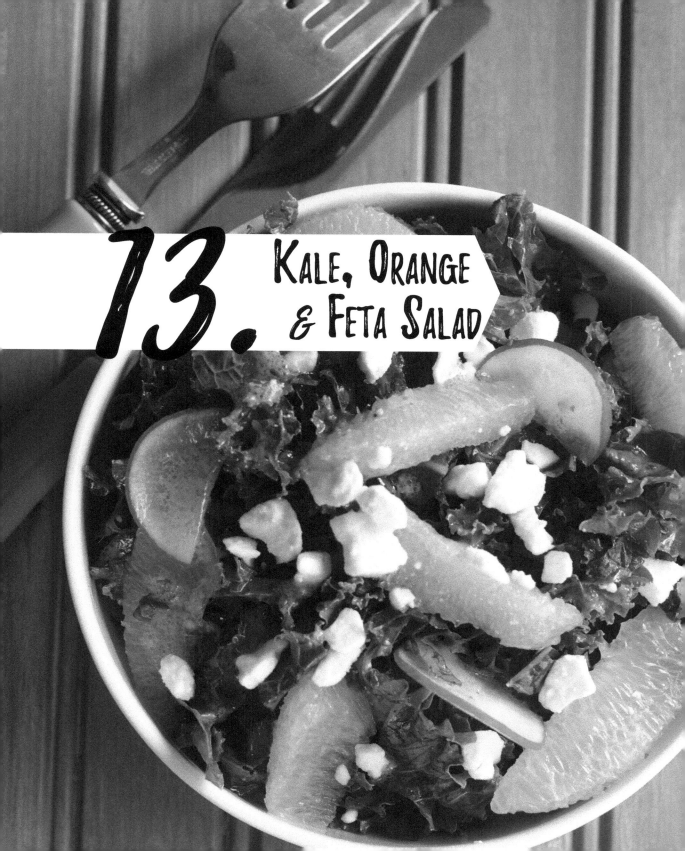

# 13.
## Kale, Orange & Feta Salad

# KALE, ORANGE, & FETA SALAD WITH CITRUS DRESSING
SERVES 2-4

 WHAT YOU NEED

## SALAD

2 cups of kale

1 teaspoon olive oil

2 tablespoons lemon juice

1 teaspoon salt

1 orange or 2-3 clementines, peeled and cut into chunks

⅓ cup crumbled feta

## DRESSING

Juice of ½ orange

1 tablespoon olive oil

½ teaspoon no sugar added dijon mustard

Pinch salt and fresh-ground pepper

¼ teaspoon orange zest

 WHAT YOU DO

1. Start by massaging the kale. To do this, first remove the stems. Then, in a large mixing bowl, combine the kale, olive oil, lemon juice and salt. With a kneading action, work to shred the kale and massage it for about three minutes or until it's soft.

2. Next, prepare the dressing. Whisk together the freshly squeezed orange juice, olive oil, dijon mustard, salt, pepper, and orange zest.

3. In a large mixing bowl, combine the kale and dressing. Then, add in the citrus fruit and top with feta cheese.

 NOTES

✓ For added flavor and nutrients, add in toasted pumpkin seeds, walnuts, pine nuts, and radishes.

Enjoy!

# 14. Chicken Pecan Grape Salad Sandwich

# CHICKEN PECAN GRAPE SALAD SANDWICH
SERVES 3-4

 WHAT YOU NEED

2 cups roasted and pulled plain chicken breast

¾ cup mayo (or to taste)

½-¾ cup grape halves

¼ cup shelled pecans

Butter lettuce leaves

8 slices of FODMAP friendly bread

Sprouts (optional)

Pinch salt and fresh-ground pepper

 WHAT YOU DO

1. Start by toasting the pecans. Heat a nonstick pan (or lightly oiled skillet) over medium-high heat. Once the pan is heated (test this with the palm of your hand 2-3 inches above the pan), reduce the heat and add the pecans. Using a wooden spoon, stir frequently so the nuts won't burn. Continue to heat until you notice the color darkening and a nutty aroma. Transfer the toasted pecans to a paper towel to cool. Once cooled, chop the nuts or lightly pulse them in a food processor until crushed.

2. Lightly toast the bread.

3. In a medium sized mixing bowl, combine the chicken, mayo, grapes, and chopped toasted pecans by mixing. Season with salt and pepper.

4. Serve equal parts of chicken salad topped with butter lettuce leaves (and sprouts if desired) between two slices of toast.

 NOTES

✓ Look for gluten-free breads that don't have honey, high fructose corn syrup, inulin, and aren't fruit-juice sweetened with high FODMAP fruit, like pear or apple.

✓ If you don't have celiac disease, you may be able to tolerate fresh sourdough bread.

✓ If possible, choose organic mayonnaise without added sugar or chemicals. Watch also for garlic, onions, and other high FODMAP ingredients.

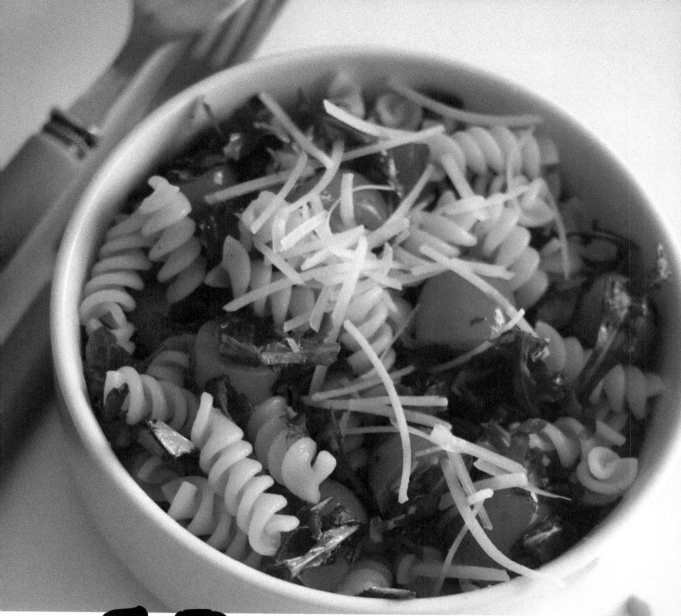

# 15. Rotini Pasta with Cherry Tomato

# Rotini Pasta with Cherry Tomato and Arugula

SERVES 2

 ## WHAT YOU NEED

8 ounces gluten-free rotini pasta

1 pint cherry tomato halves

4 tablespoons garlic-infused olive oil (Recipe #39)

1 cup arugula chopped coarsely

2-4 tablespoons chopped fresh basil

4 tablespoons shredded parmesan

Pinch coarse sea salt

 ## WHAT YOU DO

1. Start by combining the tomatoes, olive oil, arugula, basil, and sea salt in a medium sized bowl. Let ingredients sit while pasta cooks.

2. Bring a large pot of salted water to a rolling boil. Add pasta to the boiling water and let cook for seven to eight minutes (or until al dente). Stir frequently. Once the pasta is cooked, drain and quickly rinse it.

3. Add the pasta to the tomato mixture and combine ingredients by gently stirring.

4. Top with parmesan and serve warm immediately. For pasta salad, refrigerate covered for one hour. Serve cold.

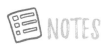 ## NOTES

*A few tips for keeping the pasta from sticking:*

✓ Make sure your water reaches a rolling boil before adding in your pasta.

✓ Stir the noodles frequently.

✓ After draining the noodles, rinse the pasta to remove excess starch.

✓ After draining, don't let the pasta sit in the colander. Serve it immediately.

✓ Add the olive oil mixture to the pasta right after you drain the noodles.

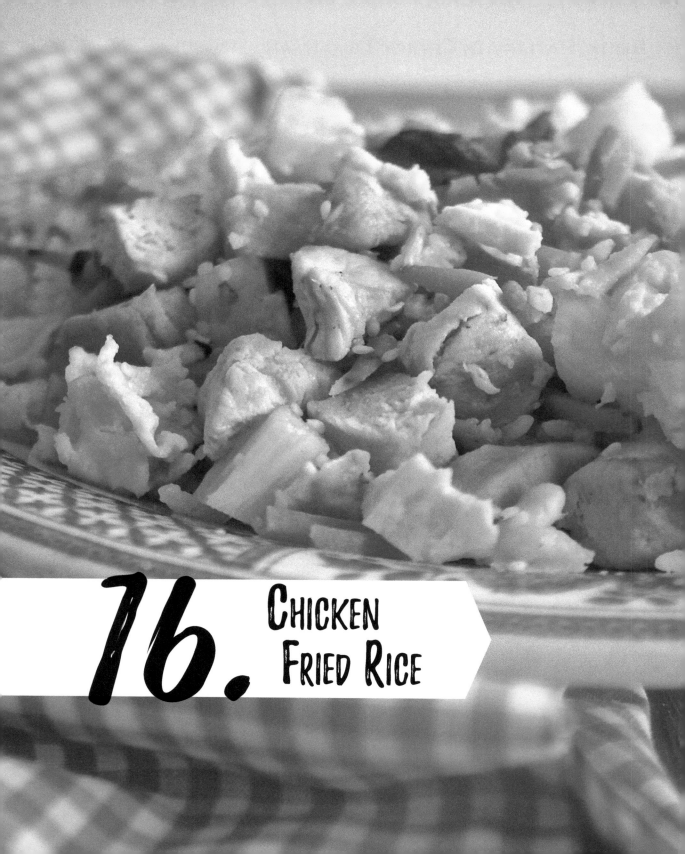

# 16. Chicken Fried Rice

# CHICKEN FRIED RICE
SERVES 4

 WHAT YOU NEED

Canola oil (enough to lightly coat the pan)

2 cups of basmati rice

2¼ cups of water

1 cup coarsely diced chicken breast

¾ cup diced pineapple

¼ cup finely diced carrots

1 egg

Sesame seeds

Pinch salt

 WHAT YOU DO

1. Start by cooking the rice. In a medium saucepan, combine the rice and water. Bring the rice to a boil. Once boiling, reduce the heat and bring the water and rice to a simmer. Cover and let cook for about 10-15 minutes. Fluff the rice with a fork.

2. Next, cook the chicken. Lightly coat a large frying pan with oil. Heat the oil over medium-high heat. Once the pan is heated (test this with the palm of your hand 2-3 inches above the pan), add diced chicken breast and sauté it until it's brown. Occasionally turn the chicken to cook evenly on each side. Season with a pinch of salt. When it's slightly browned, move chicken to the side of the pan.

3. On the opposite side of the pan, add the diced carrots and cook until they are soft.

4. In a small non-stick pan (or lightly oiled skillet), crack and scramble one egg.

5. Add the scrambled egg to the chicken and carrots and combine all of the ingredients so they are mixed. Next, add in the cooked rice and pineapple to the large frying pan. Combine all of the ingredients and sprinkle with sesame seeds and salt to taste. Serve warm.

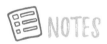 NOTES

✓ Use organic expeller-pressed canola oil, organic chicken, and organic eggs to avoid added hormones, antibiotics, pesticides, and GMOs.

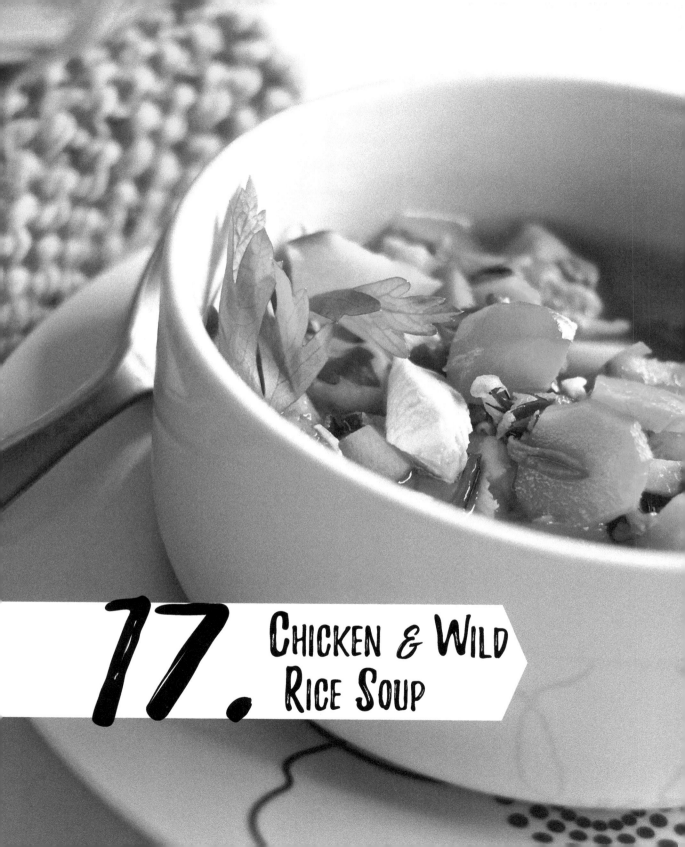

# 17. Chicken & Wild Rice Soup

# Chicken and Wild Rice Soup
Serves 4

 WHAT YOU NEED

1 tablespoon olive oil

2 cups of cubed chicken

¾ cup chopped carrots

3-4 tablespoons green onion tops

Pinch of dried thyme

2-3 tablespoons of fresh parsley

2 bay leaves

1 cup cooked wild rice

¾ cup chopped carrots

½ cup chopped zucchini

½ cup coarsely cut red pepper

5 cups low fodmap chicken or vegetable broth

Pinch sea salt and fresh-ground pepper

 WHAT YOU DO

1. In a large sauce pot, heat the olive oil. When the oil is hot (but not yet smoking), add the chicken and cook it until it's brown (about five minutes). Next, add the carrots and green onion, parsley, bay leaves, thyme, and a pinch of both salt and pepper.

2. Sauté the ingredients for about three to four minutes. Then, add the carrots, zucchini, and red peppers. Sauté all of the ingredients for about one minute.

3. Pour the stock into the pot. Raise the heat and and bring the soup to a boil. Once boiling, reduce the heat to a simmer. Allow for about five to ten minutes of simmering before adding in the cooked rice. Season with salt and pepper to taste. Garnish with fresh parsley.

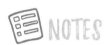 NOTES

✓ The bulbs of green onions are high FODMAP, so use only the tops.

✓ You can either freshly make the broth or purchase one. If you use store-bought, check the ingredients and avoid broths with onions or garlic.

✓ Wild rice is technically not a "rice" and has not officially been tested for FODMAPs, but I've noticed clinically that most of my patients tolerate it well. If you've got concerns about the wild rice, simply substitute brown or basmati rice instead.

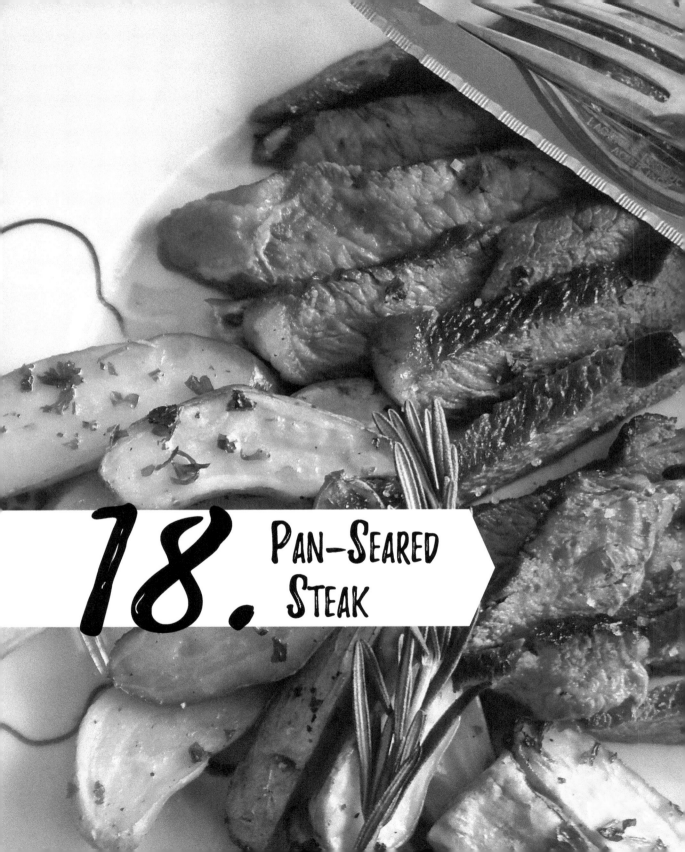

# 18. Pan-Seared Steak

# PAN-SEARED STEAK

SERVES 4

 ## WHAT YOU NEED

1½ pounds sirloin steak (cut about 1 inch thick)

1 tablespoon olive oil or canola oil

½ teaspoon sea salt

¼ teaspoon fresh-ground pepper

1-2 teaspoons dried rosemary (optional)

 ## WHAT YOU DO

1. Rub the steak with salt, pepper, and rosemary to season.
2. Heat the oil in a large skillet or frying pan over medium to medium-high heat. Once the oil is warm (test this with the palm of your hand 2-3 inches above the pan), add the seasoned meat to the pan and heat for about eight minutes on each side (for medium-temperature steak).
3. Remove from heat and let rest before slicing.

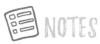 ## NOTES

✓ To avoid genetically modified ingredients, use organic expeller-pressed canola oil.

✓ Use organic beef to avoid added hormones, antibiotics, pesticides, and GMOs.

LOOKING FOR LEMON & PARSLEY FINGERLING POTATOES? LOOK NO FURTHER THAN RECIPE #33.

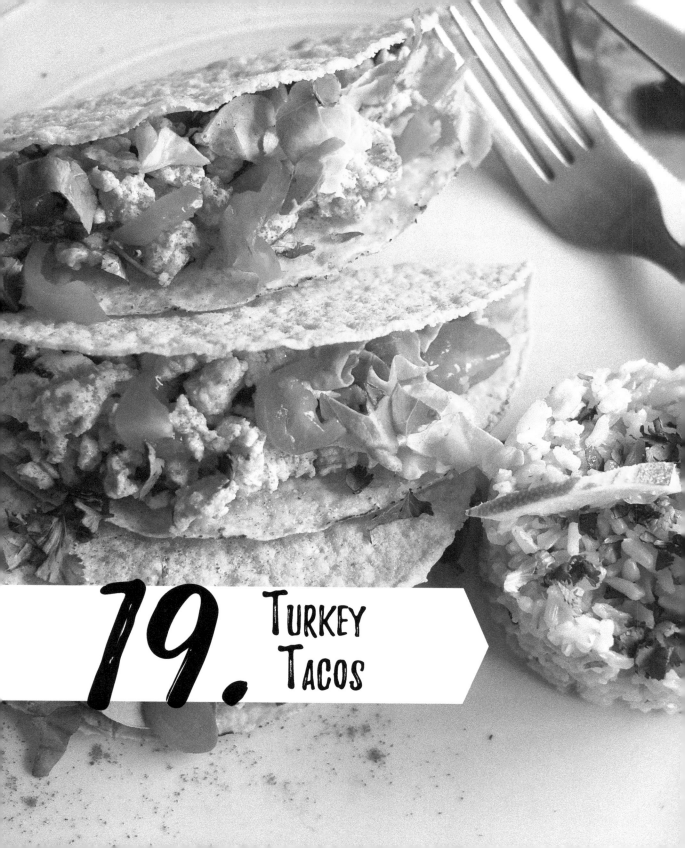

# 19. Turkey Tacos

# TURKEY TACOS
SERVES 4

 WHAT YOU NEED

8 corn taco shells

1 tablespoon canola or olive oil

1 pound ground turkey (85% lean)

Handful fresh cilantro, finely chopped

½ tablespoon chili powder

¾ teaspoon paprika

1 teaspoon salt

1 teaspoon lime zest

Juice of one lime

1 cup shredded iceberg lettuce

1 cup diced tomato

 WHAT YOU DO

1. Preheat oven to 350°F. Heat shells for 7-10 minutes or until lightly browned.
In a large mixing bowl, combine turkey, cilantro, chili powder, paprika, salt, lime zest, and lime juice. Mix ingredients together.

2. In a large skillet, heat oil. The skillet is ready when the oil is warm (test this with the palm of your hand 2-3 inches above the skillet). Add the ground turkey and break up the meat with the back of a wooden spoon. Cook until browned for 12-15 minutes.

3. Fill the taco shells with turkey, shredded lettuce, a little cilantro, and diced tomato.

 NOTES

✓ To avoid GMO ingredients and high levels of pesticides, use organic canola oil, organic corn taco shells, organic lettuce, and organic corn.

✓ Use organic ground turkey to avoid added hormones, antibiotics, pesticides, and GMOs.

LOOKING FOR CILANTRO LIME BROWN RICE? LOOK NO FURTHER THAN RECIPE #35.

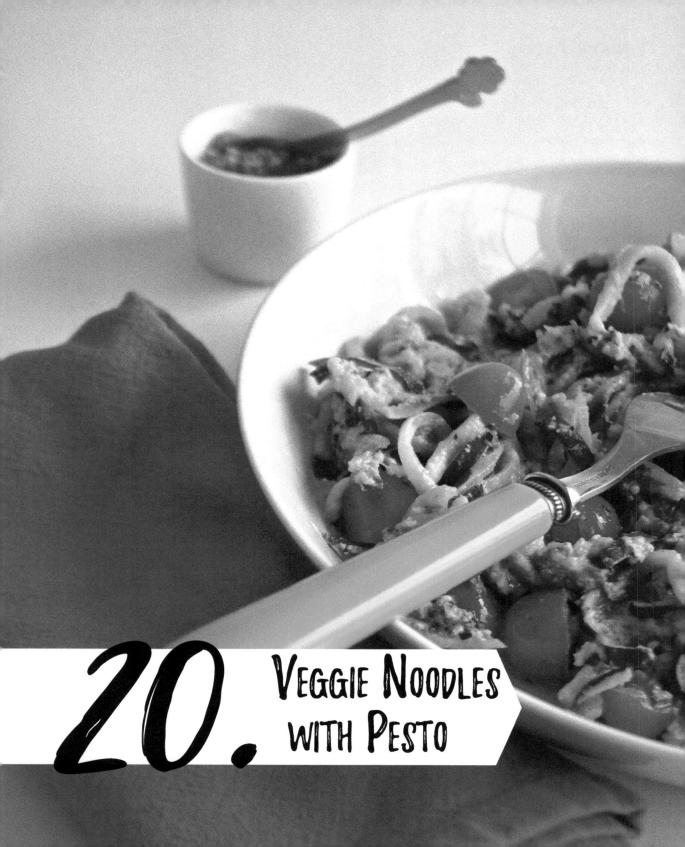

# 20. Veggie Noodles with Pesto

# VEGGIE NOODLES WITH PESTO AND CHERRY TOMATO

SERVES 4

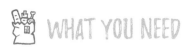 WHAT YOU NEED

## NOODLES

1 washed zucchini with skin

2 medium carrots

1 tablespoon olive oil

1 cup of cherry tomatoes, halved

## PESTO

½ cup pine nuts

1 cup basil

3-4 tablespoons olive oil

Juice of half of a lemon

Pinch salt and fresh-ground pepper

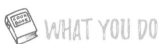 WHAT YOU DO

1. Using a mandolin, spiralizer, or julienne peeler, slice the zucchini and carrots into noodles. Then, toss the noodles with a little salt.

2. In a food processor or blender, combine the pine nuts, basil, olive oil, lemon, salt and pepper to create the pesto.

3. In a large pan, heat olive oil. The pan is ready is when the oil is warm (test this with the palm of your hand 2-3 inches above the pan). Add the carrots to the pan first and sauté for about 2 minutes. Add the zucchini to the carrots and sauté an additional 2-3 minutes.

4. Bring the heat to a low setting and add in the tomato halves and pesto. Lightly toss the ingredients. Serve Warm.

 NOTES

✓ If you're not sensitive to dairy, you can top with a little shredded mozzarella or parmesan cheese, which are both safe during elimination phase.

✓ For added flavor, use garlic-infused oil. While garlic is off limits, studies show that garlic-infused oil is safe. If you want to make your own, I've included directions with the recipe #39.

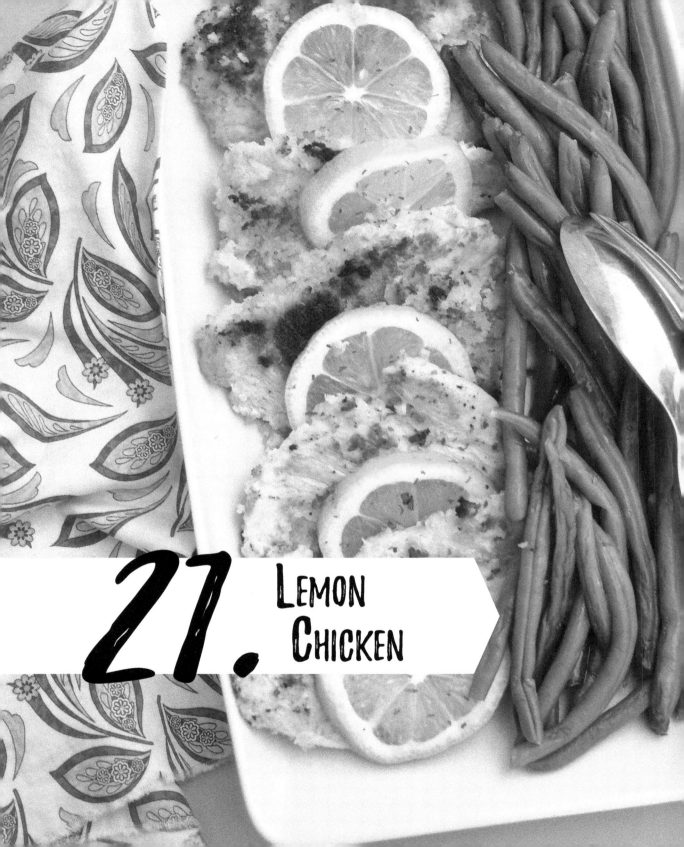

# 27.
## Lemon Chicken

# LEMON CHICKEN
SERVES 2-4

 WHAT YOU NEED

2 large skinless and boneless chicken breasts

3 eggs

2 tablespoons lemon juice

1¼ cup brown rice crumbs

1 tablespoon fresh-ground pepper

Zest of 3-4 lemons

1½ teaspoons salt

Olive oil

4 slices of lemon

 WHAT YOU DO

1. Slice the chicken breasts horizontally in half (making four pieces of chicken). Pound the chicken breasts using a meat mallet. The breasts should be about ¼" thick.

2. In a shallow bowl, combine the rice crumbs, pepper, lemon zest, and salt.

3. In another shallow bowl, beat the eggs and add in the lemon juice. Take the pounded chicken and place it into the egg/lemon mix.

4. Remove the chicken and place it into the bowl with the bread crumb mix until it's coated fully. Repeat the process until all four pieces of chicken are fully coated.

5. Coat a large skillet in a tablespoon of olive oil. Once the pan is heated (test this with the palm of your hand 2-3 inches above the pan), add the chicken breasts. Heat until fully cooked, turning once.

6. Serve with a lemon garnish.

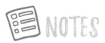 NOTES

✓ Tip: Prior to pounding, place the chicken breasts between two pieces of plastic wrap.

✓ Use organic chicken to avoid added hormones, antibiotics, pesticides and GMOs.

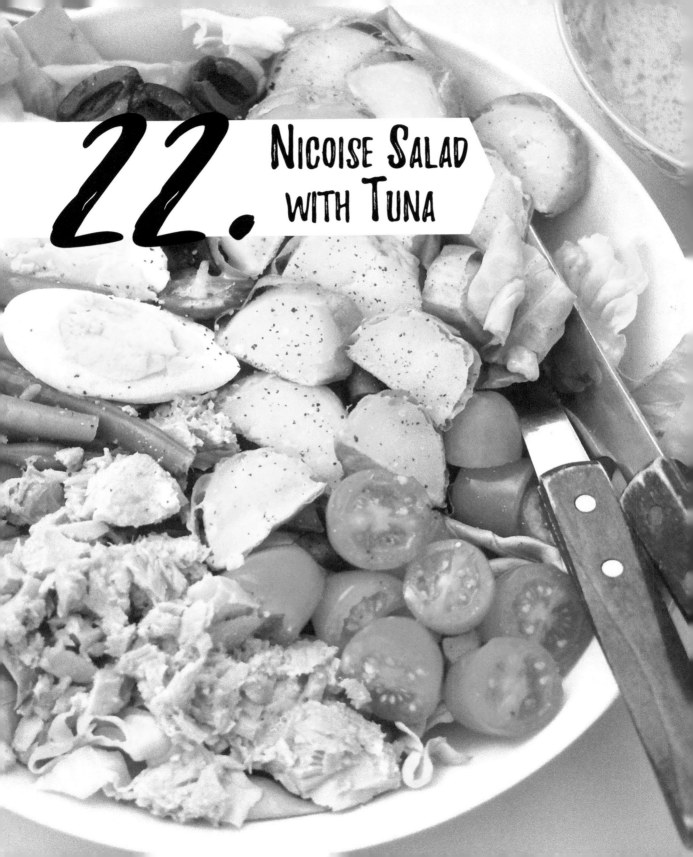

22. Nicoise Salad with Tuna

# Niçoise Salad with Tuna
## Serves 4

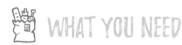 WHAT YOU NEED

### SALAD

16-20 small potatoes

½ pound trimmed haricot vert

5 cups water

20 cherry tomatoes

4 hard-boiled eggs

12 ounces of canned tuna

Pitted niçoise or kalamata olives

Bib lettuce

2 tablespoons olive oil

Pinch salt and fresh-ground pepper

### DRESSING

¼ cup olive oil

2 tablespoon fresh lemon juice

½ teaspoon fresh lemon zest

2 teaspoon dijon mustard

Pinch salt and fresh-ground pepper

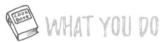 WHAT YOU DO

1. Start by preheating the oven to 450°F.
2. Prepare the dressing. In a small bowl, combine the lemon juice, zest and dijon mustard. Whisk in ¼ cup of olive oil. Season with salt and pepper to taste.
3. In a separate bowl, prepare the new potatoes for roasting by tossing them with olive oil and seasoning with salt. Place the potatoes in a single layer on a rimmed nonstick baking sheet. Roast for about 25 minutes until tender and crisp.
4. Bring water to a boil. Blanch the green beans by plunging them into a pot of boiling water for two to three minutes, then drain and rinse with ice cold water.
5. Cut olives and tomatoes into halves. Slice hard-boiled eggs into quarters.
6. Arrange vegetables, lettuce, tuna, eggs, and olives on plates or in large bowls. Drizzle with lemon vinaigrette dressing. Season with salt and pepper.

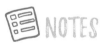 NOTES

✓ If you don't have a nonstick baking sheet, line your sheet with parchment paper.
✓ Use organic eggs to avoid added hormones, antibiotics, pesticides, and GMOs.

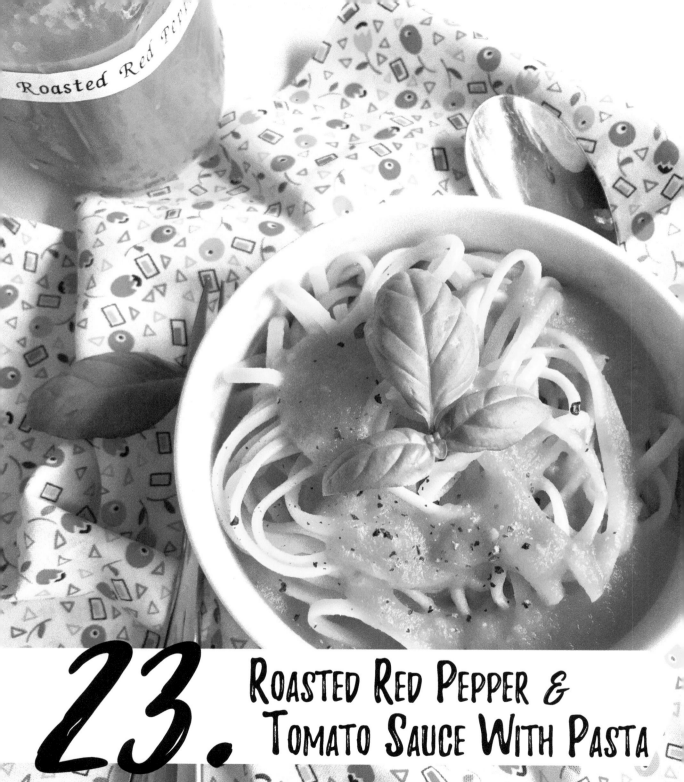

**23.** Roasted Red Pepper & Tomato Sauce With Pasta

# Roasted Red Pepper and Tomato Sauce With Pasta
## Serves 6

 WHAT YOU NEED

2 large red peppers

1-1½ pounds of tomatoes (stems removed)

1 tablespoon olive oil or garlic-infused oil

1 teaspoon dried basil

1 teaspoon dried oregano

Pinch sea salt and fresh-ground pepper

Fresh basil to taste

### SERVE WITH OPTIONS

1 pound gluten-free spaghetti (pictured)

Spaghetti squash

Veggie noodles

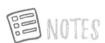 WHAT YOU DO

1. Start by preheating the oven to 450°F. Place the whole peppers and tomatoes on a rimmed baking sheet and roast on a center rack in the middle of the oven for about 30-45 minutes, turning once or twice, or until you notice a char — blackening of the outside. Remove from the oven and carefully cover with aluminum foil. Leave the tomatoes and peppers covered on the pan to cool for about 30 minutes.

2. Once cooled, remove the stems from the peppers and scoop out the seeds. You can also remove the pepper's skin (for a smoother sauce texture) by gently pulling it off. Cut the pepper into quarters. Next, cut the tomatoes into quarters.

3. Place the tomatoes and peppers in a blender or food processor. Add the olive oil, basil, oregano, and a pinch of salt and pepper. Pulse until smooth. Season with a little extra sea salt and fresh torn basil to taste and gently pulse again to stir.

4. Toss with pasta or an alternative to pasta.

 NOTES

✓ If you're not sensitive to dairy, you can top with a little shredded mozzarella or parmesan cheese.

✓ For added flavor, use garlic-infused oil. While garlic is off limits, studies show that garlic-infused oil is safe. If you want to make your own, I've included directions with recipe #39.

# 24. Stuffed Peppers

# STUFFED PEPPERS
MAKES 4

 WHAT YOU NEED

4 bell peppers

1 tablespoon olive oil

½ cup diced red pepper

½ cup diced zucchini

1 cup cooked and shredded chicken

2 cups cooked brown rice or cooked quinoa

1 tablespoon lemon juice

½ teaspoon dried oregano

½ teaspoon dried basil

½ teaspoon thyme

½ teaspoon rosemary

1 tablespoon fresh ground parsley

1 cup feta cheese

Pinch salt and fresh-ground pepper

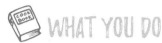 WHAT YOU DO

1. Start by preheating the oven to 350°F.
2. Next, prepare the peppers. Add water to a pot large enough to fit four peppers. Bring the water to a boil.
3. Cut the top (stem) of the pepper to remove the core and seeds. To help the pepper to stand upright, slightly trim the bottom. Place the prepared pepper into the boiling water for 3-5 minutes or until flexible. Drain in a colander and set the peppers aside.
4. Heat the oil in a large frying pan over medium-high heat. Add the zucchini and peppers. Saute for about 3-4 minutes. Next, add in the cooked chicken, cooked brown rice (or quinoa), lemon juice, herbs, spices, salt and pepper. Heat the ingredients for about 3 minutes.
5. Use a large spoon to stuff each pepper with the filling. Place the peppers filling side up into a small well oiled roasting pan. Top each pepper with ¼ cup feta cheese.
6. Roast for about 15-20 minutes or until the cheese is melted.
7. Serve warm.

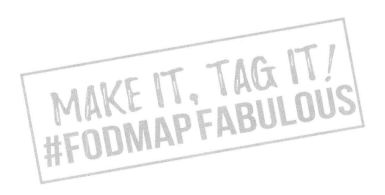

MAKE IT, TAG IT!
#FODMAPFABULOUS

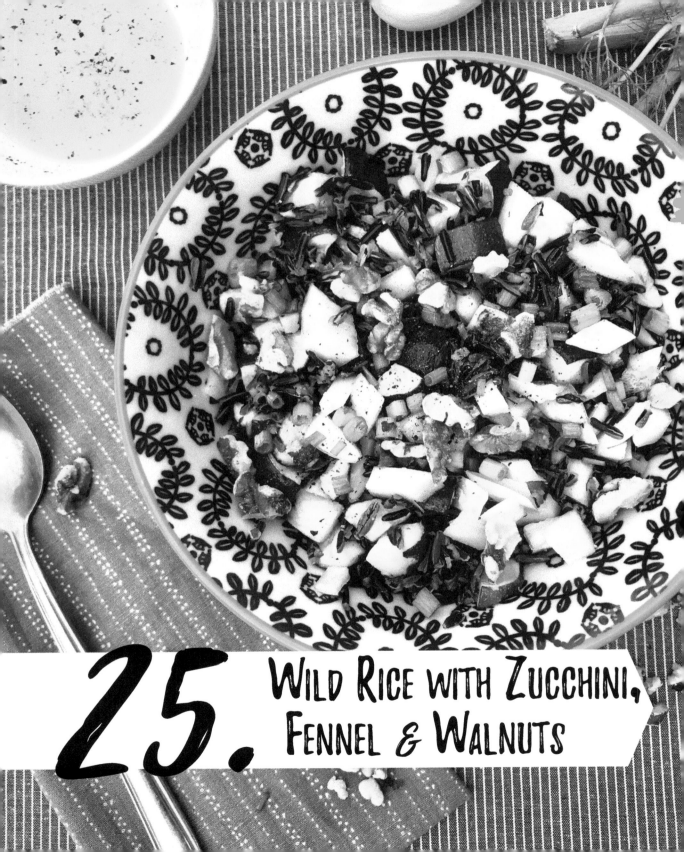

# 25. WILD RICE WITH ZUCCHINI, FENNEL & WALNUTS

# WILD RICE WITH ZUCCHINI, FENNEL, AND WALNUTS
SERVES 4

 WHAT YOU NEED

2 cups wild rice

2½ cup water

1 small zucchini

1 cup fennel bulb, diced

2-3 tablespoons sliced green onion tops

2 tablespoons of olive or walnut oil

3 tablespoons lemon juice

¾ cup walnuts

 WHAT YOU DO

1. Start by preheating the oven to 450°F.

2. In a medium saucepan, combine the rice and water. Bring the rice to a boil. Once boiling, reduce the heat and bring the water and rice to a simmer. Cover and let cook for about 10-15 minutes. Fluff the rice with a fork.

3. Coat a baking sheet with oil. Cut the zucchini quarter length into ½ inch pieces. Spread the pieces in a single layer onto the baking sheet (for added flavor, dash with salt and drizzle a little oil). Roast until moist and tender for about 10-15 minutes. Then, remove from heat and let slightly cool.

4. In a large mixing bowl, combine the rice, zucchini, diced fennel, and green onion tops.

5. In a small mixing bowl, combine oil and lemon juice. Whisk vigorously to create the dressing. Season with salt and pepper to taste. Pour the dressing over the rice mix.

6. Optional Toasted Walnuts: Heat a nonstick pan (or lightly oiled skillet) over medium-high heat. Once the pan is heated (test this with the palm of your hand 2-3 inches above the pan), reduce the heat and add the walnuts. Using a wooden spoon, stir frequently so the nuts won't burn. Continue to heat until you notice a darkening brown color and a nutty aroma. Transfer the toasted walnuts to a paper towel to cool. Once cooled, lightly chop the nuts.

7. Top the rice with walnuts and serve hot or cold.

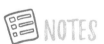 NOTES

✓ The bulbs of green onions are high fodmap, so use only the tops.

✓ Wild rice is technically not a "rice" and has not officially been tested for FODMAPs, but I've noticed clinically that most of my patients tolerate it well. If you've got concerns about the wild rice, simply substitute brown or basmati rice instead.

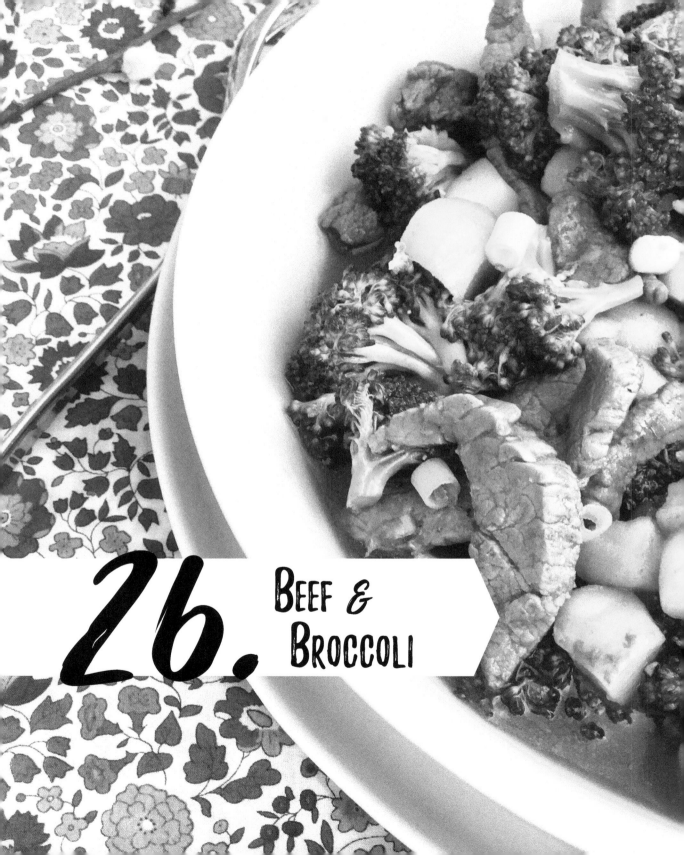

26.

Beef &
Broccoli

# BEEF AND BROCCOLI
## SERVES 4

 WHAT YOU NEED

¾ pound top round steak

2 cups broccoli florets (heads only)

10 ounce can sliced water chestnuts

½ cup green onion tops

2 teaspoons canola oil or olive oil

## SAUCE

½ cup low FODMAP broth

3 tablespoons soy sauce

1 tablespoon cornstarch

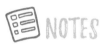 WHAT YOU DO

1. Slice steak into ¼ inch strips about 2 inches long. Cut asparagus into 1-inch pieces. Drain water chestnuts.
2. Mix together broth, soy sauce, and cornstarch.
3. In a wok or large large frying pan, heat the oil over medium-high heat. Add the steak and cook for about 2-3 minutes. Add the asparagus, water chestnuts, and green onion tops and cook for another 4-5 minutes or until the vegetables are tender.
4. With a wooden spoon, stir in the sauce. Cook and gently stir the ingredients until all ingredients are fully cooked.

NOTES

✓ Serve with rice or rice noodles.

✓ To avoid added hormones, antibiotics, pesticides and GMOs, use organic beef.

✓ To avoid GMOs, use organic cornstarch and expeller-pressed canola oil.

✓ Read soy sauce labels carefully and avoid high-fructose corn syrup.

✓ To keep it low FODMAP, eat only 1 cup (or less) of broccoli florets per meal.

✓ You can either freshly make the broth or purchase one. If you use store-bought, check the ingredients and avoid broths with onions and/or garlic.

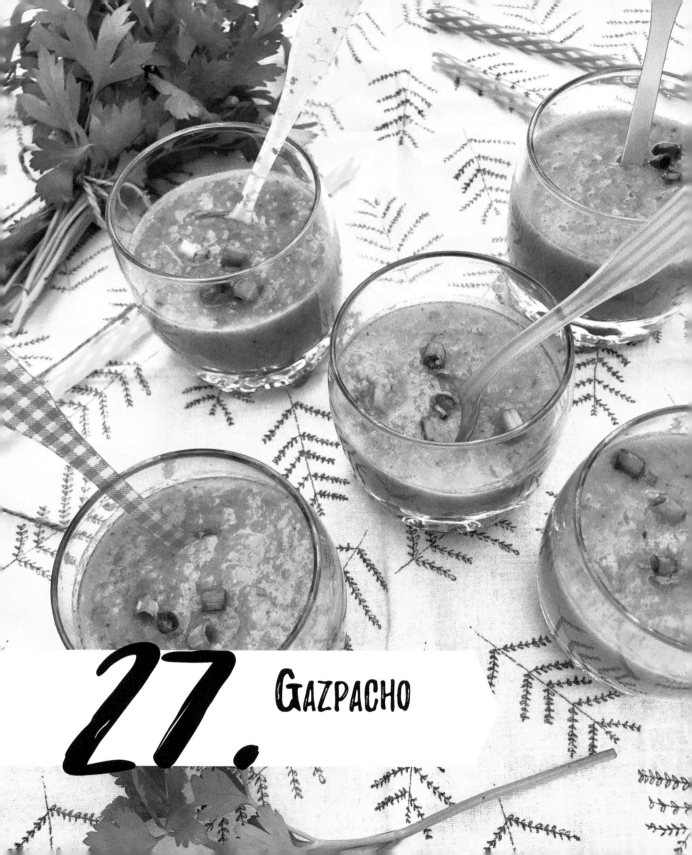

# 27. Gazpacho

# GAZPACHO
SERVES 4-6

 WHAT YOU NEED

6 ripe tomatoes

½ red pepper

½ yellow pepper

1 small cucumber

6 thin green onions (tops only)

½ cup chilled low FODMAP broth

½ cup chilled tomato juice

## DRESSING

2 tablespoons lemon juice

6 tablespoons olive oil

2-3 tablespoons fresh-chopped parsley

2-3 tablespoons fresh-chopped basil

½ teaspoon salt

Pepper to taste

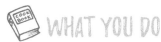 WHAT YOU DO

1. Start by prepping the vegetables. Slice the ripe tomatoes into small pieces and remove the seeds. Deseed and dice the peppers. Peel and cut the cucumber into small pieces. Cut the green onions into thin slices (reserve a few on the side for garnish). Place the tomatoes, peppers, cucumber, and green onions in a large mixing bowl.

2. In a smaller mixing bowl, combine the lemon juice, olive oil, salt, and pepper by vigorously whisking. Stir in the basil and parsley.

3. Pour the dressing over the prepared vegetables, combine gently with a spoon, and place the bowl in the refrigerator for at least two hours.

4. Remove the bowl from the fridge and stir in the cold broth and tomato juice just before serving. Garnish with green onion tops. Serve chilled.

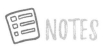 NOTES

✓ You can either freshly make the broth or purchase one. If you use store-bought, check the ingredients and avoid broths with onions, garlic, or other high FODMAP ingredients.

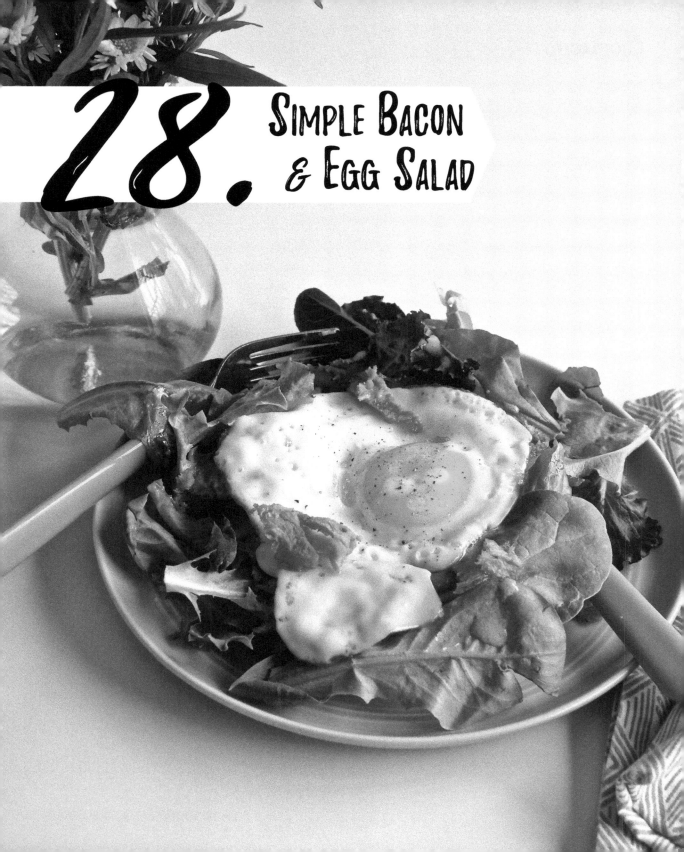

# 28.
## Simple Bacon & Egg Salad

# SIMPLE BACON AND EGG SALAD

SERVES 4

 WHAT YOU NEED

## SALAD

8 slices of turkey bacon

6 cups mesclun greens

4 teaspoons olive oil

4 eggs

Salt and pepper to taste

## DRESSING

⅓ cup olive oil

¼ cup cider vinegar

1 tablespoon dijon mustard

½ teaspoon salt

¼ teaspoon fresh-ground pepper

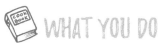 WHAT YOU DO

1. Start by frying your eggs. Place a large frying pan over medium heat and add olive oil. Swirl olive oil in the pan to evenly coat the surface, using one teaspoon of olive oil per egg. The pan is ready is when the oil is warm (test this with the palm of your hand 2-3 inches above the pan). Next, crack the egg directly into the skillet. Let it cook without moving it. The whites will start to set after a few minutes (followed by the yolk). Cover the pan part way through cooking. The steam from the egg and oil will set the top. You'll know it's done when the whites are set and the yolk is thickened. Season with salt and pepper.

2. Bake the bacon by placing it in a single layer in a large shallow baking pan. Bake at 375-400°F to desired crispness (about 16-19 minutes). Once the bacon is crispy, remove it from the oven and place it between two paper towels to reduce moisture. Chop the bacon into thin bits.

3. Make the dressing. In a mixing bowl, briskly whisk together the olive oil, cider vinegar, dijon mustard, salt, and pepper.

4. Place the greens in a large bowl and toss them with dressing (measured to taste). Add equal amounts of dressed salad to four bowls. Top the greens with chopped bacon bits and a fried egg.

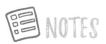 NOTES

✓ Look for bacon that is free from nitrates/nitrites, chemicals, garlic or onion, and added sugar.

✓ Look for a dijon mustard without added sugar, onion, or garlic powder.

✓ Use organic eggs to avoid added hormones, antibiotics, pesticides and GMOs.

✓ Poached eggs can be used in place of fried.

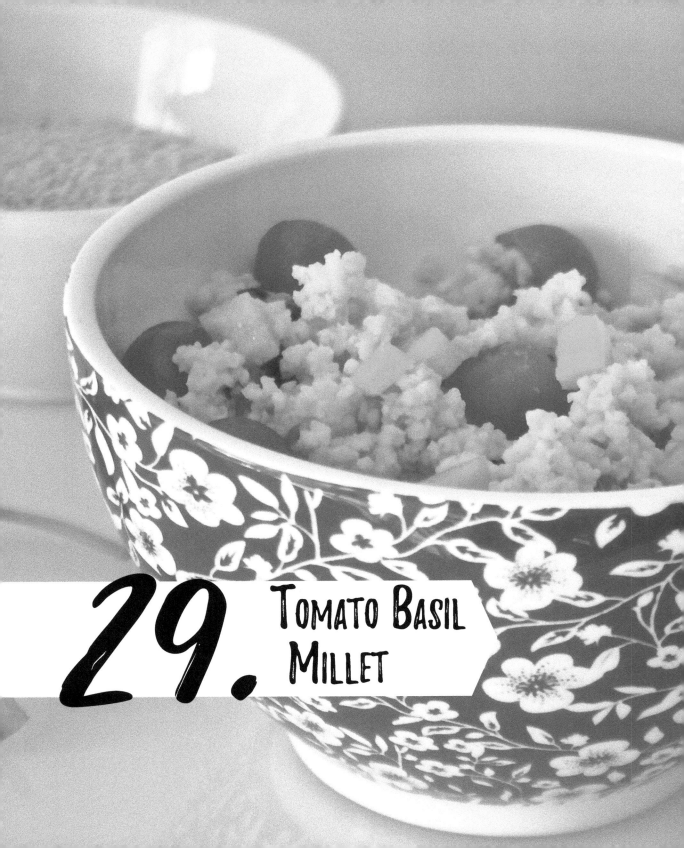

# 29.
## Tomato Basil Millet

# TOMATO BASIL MILLET

 WHAT YOU NEED

1 cup uncooked millet

2 cups water

30 grape tomatoes

½ yellow bell pepper diced

¼ cup basil leaves

3 tablespoons olive oil

Sea salt to taste

 WHAT YOU DO

1. Add millet to a dry saucepan. Toast the millet for about four minutes over medium heat. Add in the water and a pinch of salt. Bring to a boil, then reduce the heat to low and cover.

2. Simmer for about 15 minutes or until the liquid is absorbed. Remove from heat and let it sit covered for about 10 minutes.

3. Use a paring knife to slice the tomatoes in half, dice the yellow pepper, and julienne (cut into matchstick thin slices) the basil.

4. In a large bowl, combine the tomato, pepper, basil, and olive oil. Add the millet to the mixture and gently combine. Season with sea salt to taste.

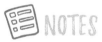 NOTES

✓ For added flavor, substitute the traditional olive oil with garlic (see recipe #39) or basil-infused olive oil.

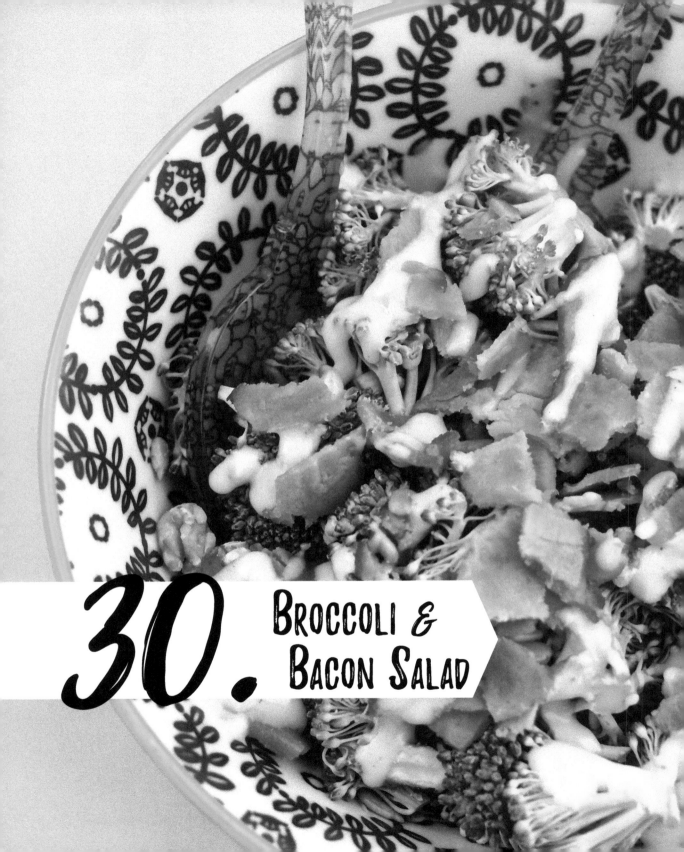

# 30.
## Broccoli &
## Bacon Salad

# BROCCOLI AND BACON SALAD
SERVES 4-6

 WHAT YOU NEED

2 heads broccoli florets (heads only)

⅓ cup mayonnaise

2 tablespoons pure maple syrup

1 tablespoon apple cider vinegar

¼ cup walnuts (chopped)

2 tablespoons roasted and salted sunflower seeds

½ tablespoons salt

¼ teaspoon fresh-ground pepper

6-8 slices bacon or turkey bacon

 WHAT YOU DO

1. Start by preparing the bacon. Bake the bacon by placing it in a single layer on a large, shallow baking pan. Bake at 375-400°F to desired crispness (about 16-19 minutes). Once the bacon is crispy, remove it from the oven and place it between two paper towels to reduce moisture. Chop the bacon into thin bits.

2. In a small mixing bowl, whisk together mayonnaise, maple syrup, vinegar, salt, and pepper to make the dressing.

3. Combine broccoli, seeds, walnuts, and cooked bacon in a separate large bowl.

4. Add the dressing to the large bowl and mix well. Season with salt and pepper.

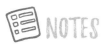 NOTES

✓ Look for bacon that is free from nitrates and nitrites, chemicals, garlic or onions, and added sugar.

✓ If possible, choose organic mayonnaise without added sugar or chemicals. Watch also for garlic, onions, and other high FODMAP ingredients.

✓ To keep it low FODMAP, eat only 1 cup (or less) of broccoli florets per meal. Find it hard to eat broccoli raw? Try it blanched! See page 50 for details.

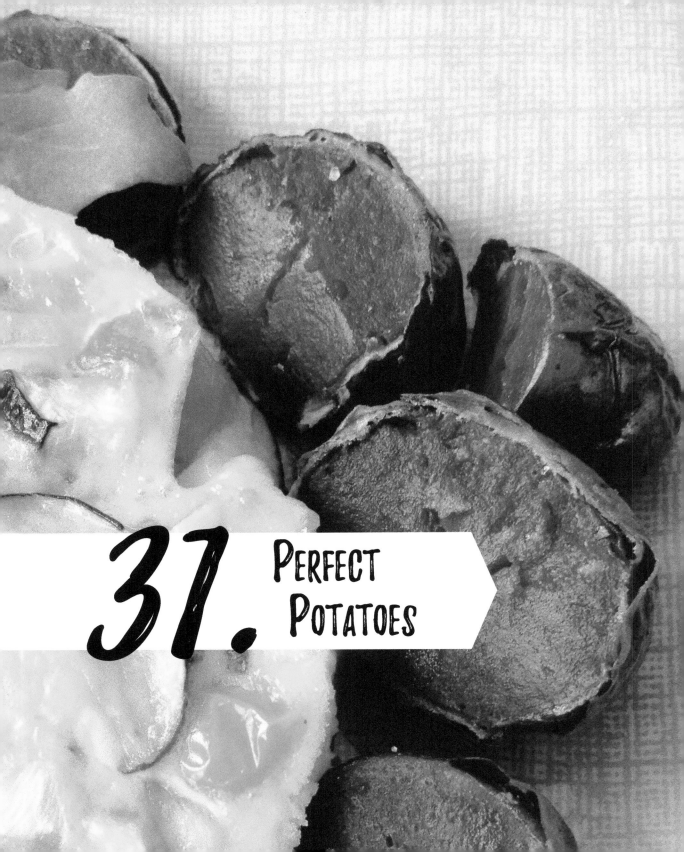

# 37. Perfect Potatoes

# PERFECT POTATOES
SERVES 4-6

 ## WHAT YOU NEED

6-8 purple potatoes

1 tablespoon olive oil

⅛ teaspoon sea salt

1 tablespoon dried rosemary (optional)

 ## WHAT YOU DO

1. Start by preheating the oven to 450°F.
2. Cut potatoes in half. Then, cut them in half again. Toss the cut potatoes with a tablespoon of olive oil. Add a dash of sea salt and a tablespoon of dried rosemary.
3. Transfer the potatoes to a baking sheet. Roast them for about 45-60 minutes until they are crispy at the edges and tender in the middle. Use a spatula to flip the potatoes twice while they're roasting to ensure even cooking.
4. Serve while hot and crispy.

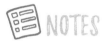 ## NOTES

✓ Feel free to substitute the purple potatoes with red, brown or white.

✓ Sweet potatoes in a quantity greater than ½ cup are considered high fodmap.

✓ For precise measurement, a dash is equal to ⅛ teaspoon.

LOOKING FOR FRITTATA? LOOK NO FURTHER THAN RECIPE #2.

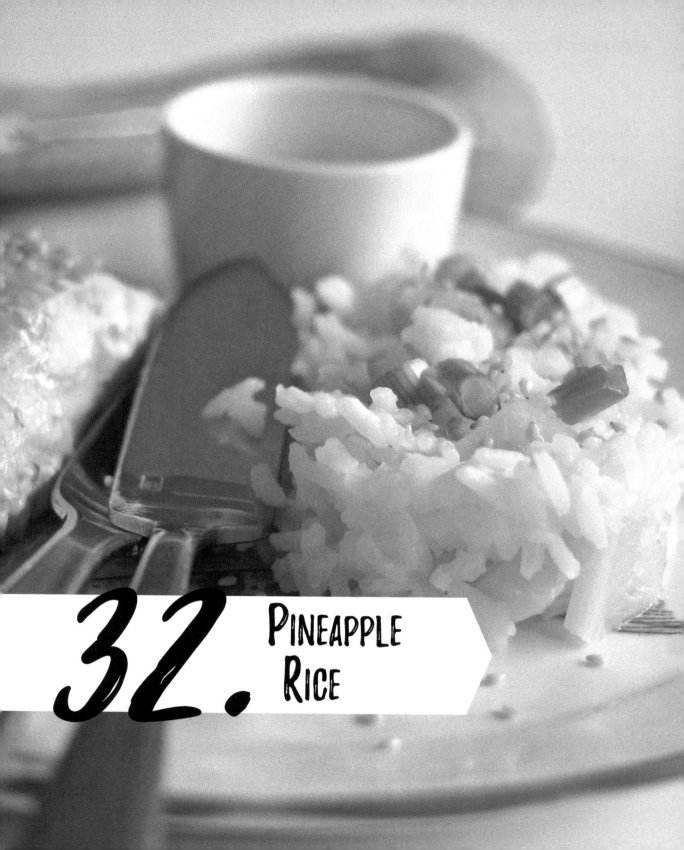

# 32. Pineapple Rice

# PINEAPPLE RICE

 ## WHAT YOU NEED

2 cups basmati rice

2¼ cups water

½ cup diced pineapple

4 tablespoons green onion tops (optional)

Toasted sesame seeds

Salt to taste

 ## WHAT YOU DO

1. In a medium saucepan, combine the rice and water. Bring the rice to a boil. Once boiling, reduce the heat and bring the water and rice to a simmer. Cover and let cook for about 10-15 minutes. Fluff the rice with a fork.

2. In a large mixing bowl, combine the cooked rice, diced pineapple, and green onion tops. Sprinkle the dish with toasted sesame seeds and salt to taste.

 ## NOTES

✓ Basmati rice can be substituted with brown or wild rice for added nutrients.

✓ To add more sesame flavor, drizzle with sesame oil.

LOOKING FOR SOY, SESAME MAPLE SALMON? LOOK NO FURTHER THAN RECIPE #12.

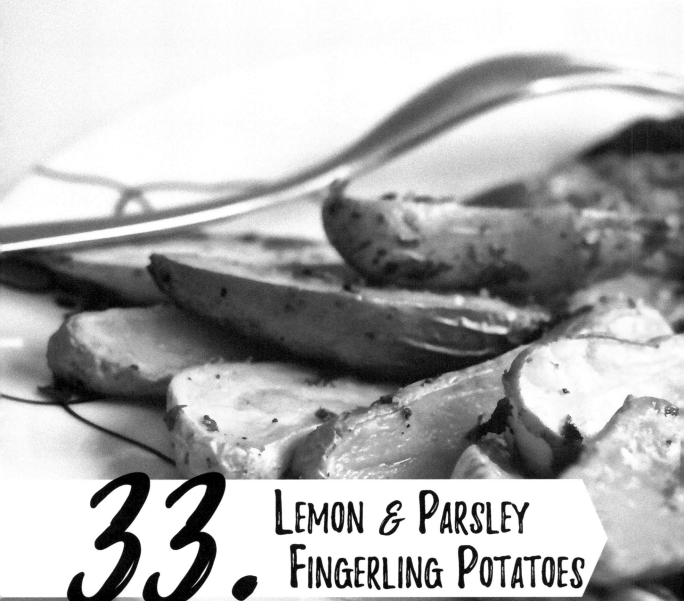

**33.** Lemon & Parsley Fingerling Potatoes

# LEMON AND PARSLEY FINGERLING POTATOES

SERVES 4

 WHAT YOU NEED

1 pound of fingerling potatoes

2 tablespoons olive oil

2 tablespoons fresh-squeezed lemon juice

2 tablespoons fresh-chopped flat-leaf parsley

½ tablespoon salt

1 tablespoon fresh lemon zest

Fresh-ground Himalayan sea salt to taste

 WHAT YOU DO

1. Preheat the oven to 450°F.

2. Cut fingerling potatoes in half, lengthwise.

3. In a large mixing bowl, toss potatoes, olive oil, lemon juice, parsley, and salt.

4. Next, transfer the potatoes to a shallow, lightly oiled baking sheet and roast for about 35-40 minutes until golden. Occasionally turn the potatoes to ensure even cooking. Remove from the oven when browned and sprinkle with lemon zest and sea salt. Serve hot or cold.

 NOTES

✓ If Himalayan sea salt is unavailable, substitute with any sea salt. Sea salt is a rich source of trace minerals and is a healthier alternative to traditional table salt.

LOOKING FOR PAN-SEARED STEAK? LOOK NO FURTHER THAN RECIPE #18.

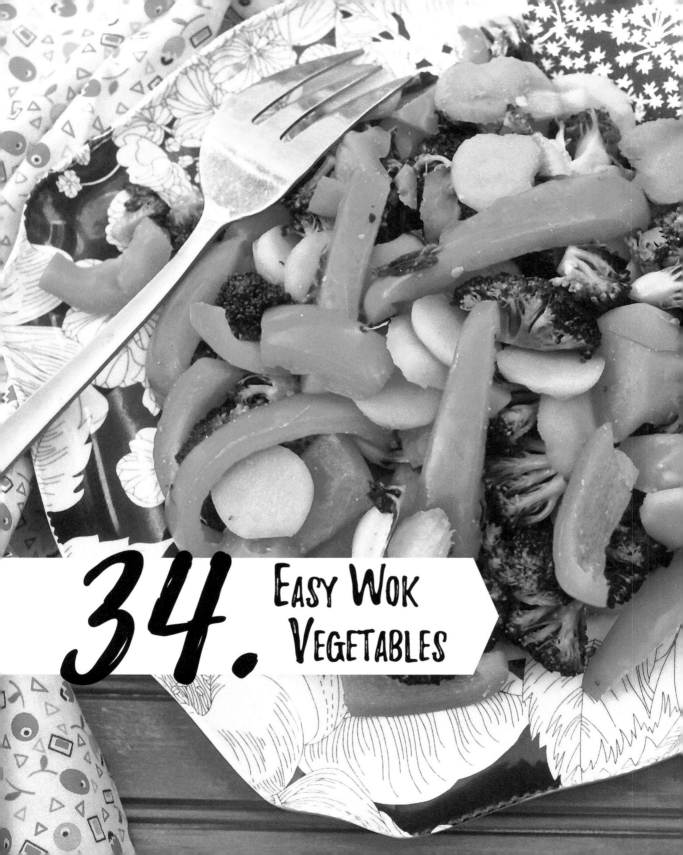

# 34. Easy Wok Vegetables

# EASY WOK VEGETABLES
SERVES 4-6

 WHAT YOU NEED

1 tablespoon toasted sesame oil

2 cups broccoli florets, heads only

1 cup sliced water chestnuts

1 red bell pepper, cut into thin slices

4 bunches baby bok choy, chopped into large pieces

¼ cup pineapple juice

1 tablespoon minced ginger

2 tablespoons tamari

Optional: 6-8 tablespoons of peanuts, dry-roasted and chopped

 WHAT YOU DO

1. Start by heating the oil In a wok or large sauté pan on medium-high heat.

2. Once the oil is warm (test this with the palm of your hand 2-3 inches above the pan), add broccoli, water chestnuts, red bell peppers, and baby bok choy. With a wooden spoon, stir frequently for three minutes or until veggies begin to stick to the pan.

3. Add pineapple juice to deglaze the pan, then stir in the ginger and tamari. Continue to cook on medium-high heat until the veggies are tender but still crispy.

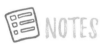 NOTES

✓ If you experience juice sensitivity, substitute the pineapple juice with water.

✓ To keep it low FODMAP, eat only 1 cup (or less) of broccoli florets per meal.

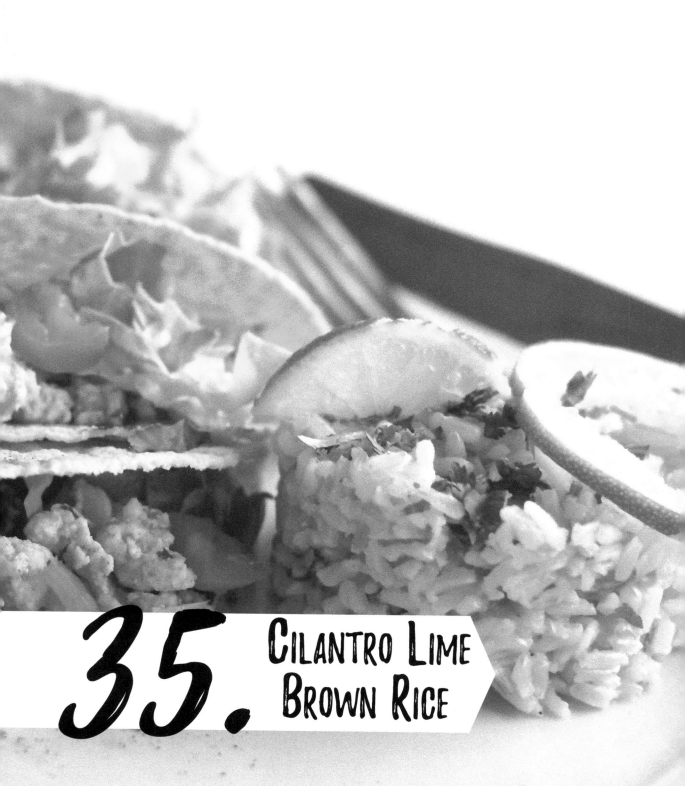

**35.** Cilantro Lime Brown Rice

# Cilantro Lime Brown Rice

SERVES 4

## WHAT YOU NEED

2 cups brown rice

2 ¼ cup water

½ lime, juice and zest

2-4 tablespoons chopped cilantro

1 tablespoon canola or olive oil

¼ teaspoon salt

## WHAT YOU DO

1. In a medium saucepan, combine the rice and water. Bring the rice to a boil. Once boiling, reduce the heat and bring the water and rice to a simmer. Cover and let cook for about 10-15 minutes. Fluff the rice with a fork.

2. In a large mixing bowl, combine the rice, lime juice and zest, cilantro, oil and salt. Serve warm.

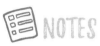

## NOTES

✓ Brown rice can be substituted with basmati or wild rice.

✓ To avoid genetically modified ingredients, use organic canola oil.

LOOKING FOR TACOS? LOOK NO FURTHER THAN RECIPE #19.

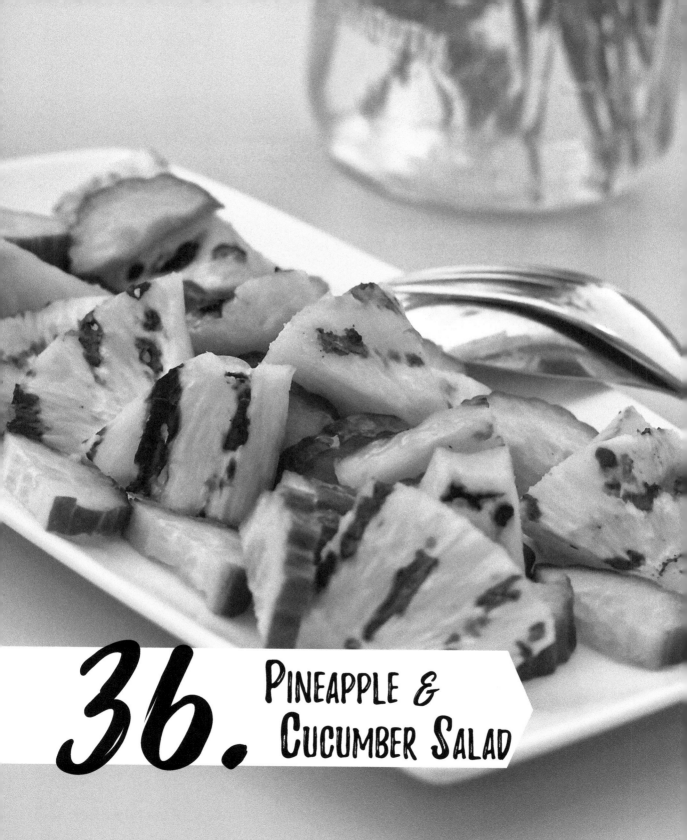

# 36. Pineapple & Cucumber Salad

# PINEAPPLE AND CUCUMBER SALAD

SERVES 4

 ## WHAT YOU NEED

1 pineapple cored and cut into thick rings

1 large English cucumber

1 tablespoon olive oil

2 limes, zest and juice

½ teaspoon coarse sea salt

 ## WHAT YOU DO

1. Start by brushing the pineapple with a little olive oil. Place the pineapple rounds onto a heated grill until grill marks appear (about two minutes per side). Remove the pineapple from the grill and let it cool.

2. Cut the pineapple into large bits.

3. Slice the cucumber into rounds, then cut rounds in half.

4. In a large mixing bowl, combine and evenly mix the pineapple, cucumber, olive oil, lime juice, lime zest and than season with sea salt. Serve immediately or chill the fridge.

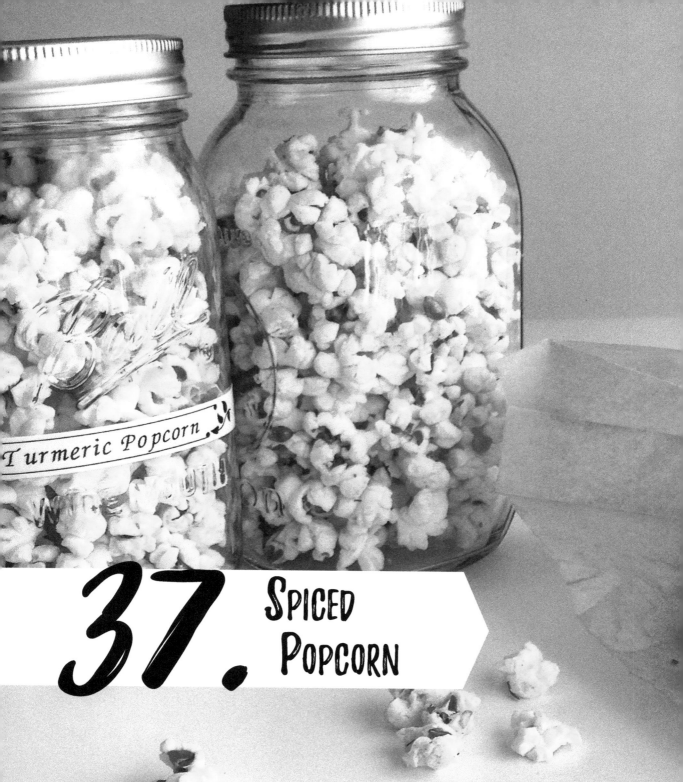

Turmeric Popcorn

# 37. SPICED POPCORN

# SPICED POPCORN
SERVES 4

 ## WHAT YOU NEED

3 tablespoons canola, avocado, or sesame oil

½ cup unpopped corn kernels

½-1 teaspoon turmeric

½ teaspoon salt

### Optional Additions

2 tablespoons pure maple syrup

¼ teaspoon or pinch of cayenne pepper

2 tablespoons toasted sesame seeds

 ## WHAT YOU DO

1. In a large pot, heat 2 tablespoons of oil over high heat for 45 seconds to one minute. Add the kernels to the pot and place the lid tightly on top. Reduce the heat to medium and shake the pot to ensure that all kernels get evenly coated.

2. Listen closely, and once you hear the popcorn slowing to a few pops every few seconds, remove from heat.

3. Gently stir in the remaining ingredients and desired additions.

 ## NOTES

✓ Store in an airtight container for up to three days.

✓ To avoid GMO ingredients and high levels of pesticides, use organic canola oil and organic corn.

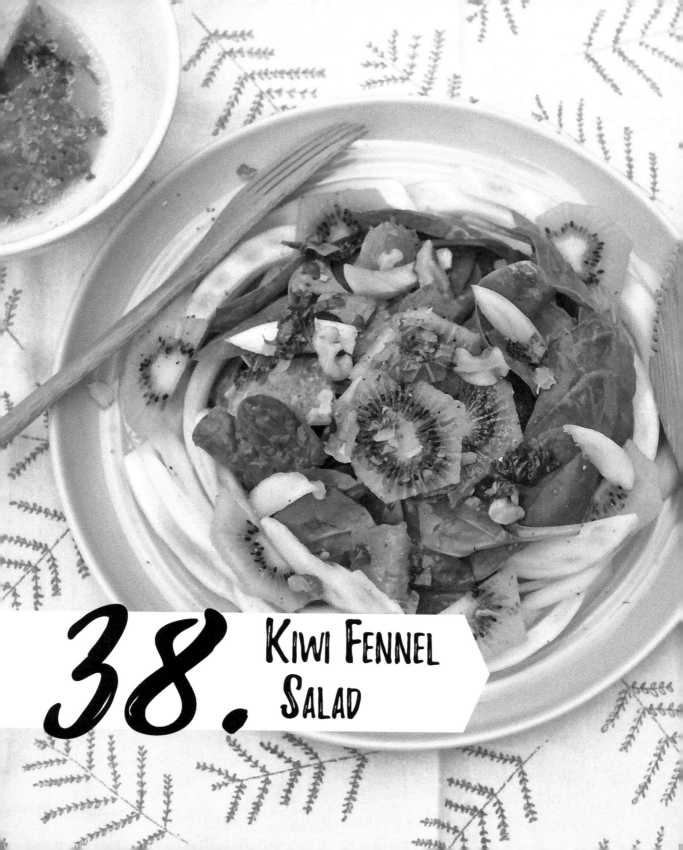

# 38. Kiwi Fennel Salad

# KIWI FENNEL SALAD
SERVES 4

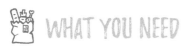 WHAT YOU NEED

## SALAD

¼ cup shelled walnuts

6 kiwis

1 small fennel bulb

6 cups spinach

2 oranges

## ORANGE AND MINT DRESSING

2 oranges

1-2 tablespoons fresh, chopped mint

1 ½ tablespoons rice wine vinegar

¾ cup olive oil

Salt and fresh-ground pepper to taste

 WHAT YOU DO

1. Start by toasting the walnuts. Heat a nonstick pan (or lightly oiled skillet) over medium-high heat. Once the pan is heated (test this with the palm of your hand 2-3 inches above the pan), reduce the heat and add the walnuts. Using a wooden spoon, stir frequently so the nuts won't burn. Continue to heat until you notice a darkening and a nutty aroma. Transfer the toasted walnuts to a paper towel to cool. Once cooled, lightly chop the nuts.

2. Wash and cut the kiwi. Using a sharp fruit knife, cut the kiwi in half down the middle. Using a spoon, scoop the fruit out from the skin. Dice the fruit into large cubes.

3. Scrub the fennel bulb. Cut off the stalk (stems and fronds) — you can either save these for another recipe or discard. Cut off the bottom (root end) and discard. Remove the tough core from the middle and place the bulb cut side down on a cutting board. Use a sharp knife to slice the bulb lengthwise into thin strips.

4. Peel the orange and cut slices in half.

5. For the dressing, add all of the ingredients to a jar with a tightly fitting lid. Shake until fully combined.

6. In a large serving bowl, place the spinach at the bottom. Add the fennel, then layer the kiwis and the oranges. Top with the toasted walnuts and dressing.

 NOTES

✓ If for any reason you don't tolerate vinegar, you can just omit it from the dressing.

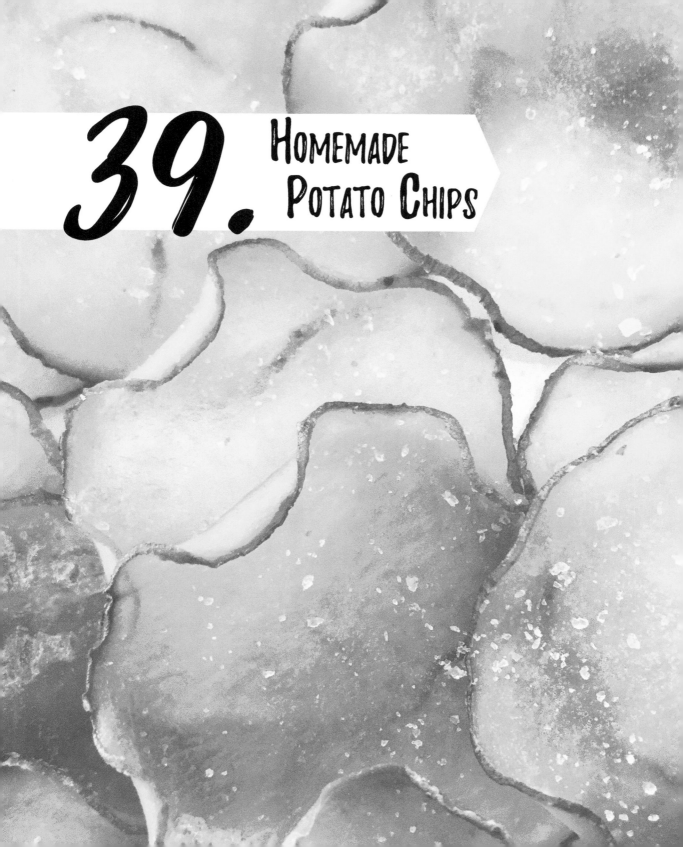

# 39. Homemade Potato Chips

# HOMEMADE POTATO CHIPS

SERVES 4

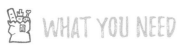 WHAT YOU NEED

4 medium-sized potatoes

½ teaspoon coarse salt

## GARLIC-INFUSED OLIVE OIL

1 cup olive oil

5-6 peeled cloves of garlic

4 tablespoons garlic-infused olive oil

Parchment paper

 WHAT YOU DO

1. To begin, preheat your oven to 400°F. Prepare two rimmed baking sheets by lightly coating them with olive oil.

2. **To make the garlic-infused oil:** While garlic is notoriously high FODMAP, garlic oil is considered safe. If for any reason you don't tolerate garlic oil, you can use plain olive oil. Add the garlic and oil to a small saucepan over high heat. Bring the oil to a boil. Once boiling, reduce the heat to low and let simmer for about three to five minutes. Over cooking the garlic will make it bitter. Once the garlic is lightly browned, remove the pot from the heat and let it rest for about five minutes. Once cooled, strain the garlic from the oil. You'll need about 3-4 tablespoons for this recipe. The remaining oil is good for two to three days, but it must be stored in the fridge in a glass airtight container. The oil is only safe to use for up to three days after you make it.

3. Using a mandolin or sharp knife, slice the potatoes into ¼ inch thick slices.

4. In a large mixing bowl, toss to combine the potato slices, olive oil, and salt.

5. Place the potato slices in a single layer onto the prepared baking sheets. Put the sheets into the oven for 20 minutes (or until crisp), rotating after 10 minutes.

6. Remove from the oven and transfer the potatoes onto the parchment paper. Sprinkle with salt and let dry.

 NOTES

✓ If you need an alternative for garlic-infused oil, use pure olive oil instead.

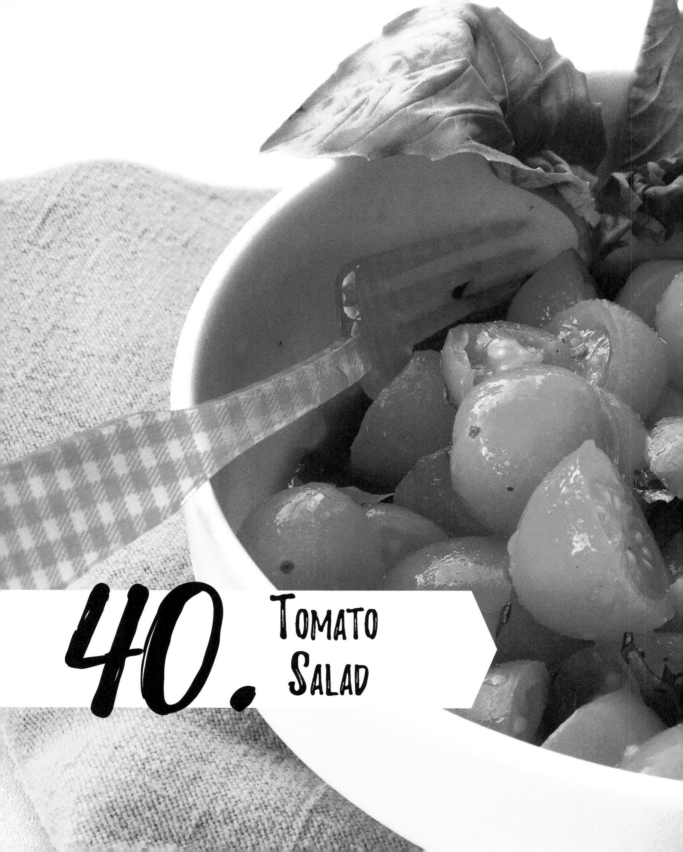

# 40.
## Tomato Salad

# TOMATO SALAD
SERVES 4

 ## WHAT YOU NEED

1 quart cherry tomatoes cut in half

¼ cup olive oil

2-3 tablespoons balsamic vinegar

½ teaspoon salt

1-2 tablespoons fresh-chopped parsley

1-2 tablespoons fresh-chopped basil

¼ teaspoon dried oregano

Pepper to taste

Extra basil for added flavor and garnish

 ## WHAT YOU DO

1. Start by making the dressing. In a mixing bowl, combine the olive oil, vinegar, salt, parsley, basil, oregano, and pepper. Whisk vigorously.

2. Place the cherry tomato halves in a large serving bowl. Toss the tomatoes with the dressing (to taste). Season with salt and pepper to taste. Add in some freshly torn basil.

3. Cover and refrigerate for three to four hours or overnight prior to serving.

# 47. Deviled Eggs

# Deviled Eggs

MAKES 12 DEVILED EGGS

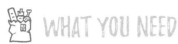 WHAT YOU NEED

6 hard boiled eggs

¼ cup of mayonnaise

¼-½ teaspoon mustard powder or 1 tablespoon prepared mustard

Salt and fresh-ground pepper to taste

Pinch paprika

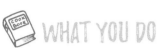 WHAT YOU DO

1. Start by hard-boiling your eggs. First, place the eggs at the bottom of a saucepan or pot. Next, add cold water until the eggs are fully covered by about 2 inches, then add a pinch of salt to the water.  Bring the water to a rolling boil. Once it's boiling, turn off the heat and cover the pot. Let the eggs sit for about 12-15 minutes. Carefully strain the hot water from the pot and run the eggs under cold water. Next, peel the eggs.

2. Once the eggs are peeled, cut each egg lengthwise and gently remove the yolk. In a small mixing bowl, combine the yolk, mayo, mustard powder, salt, and pepper. You can either mix by hand or by using a food processor or immersion blender.

3. Scoop the mixture evenly back into each egg half. Sprinkle with paprika. If desired, garnish with fresh herbs.

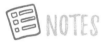 NOTES

✓ Use organic eggs to avoid added hormones, antibiotics, pesticides and GMOs.

✓ If possible, choose organic mayonnaise without added sugar or chemicals. Watch for garlic, onions, and other high FODMAP ingredients.

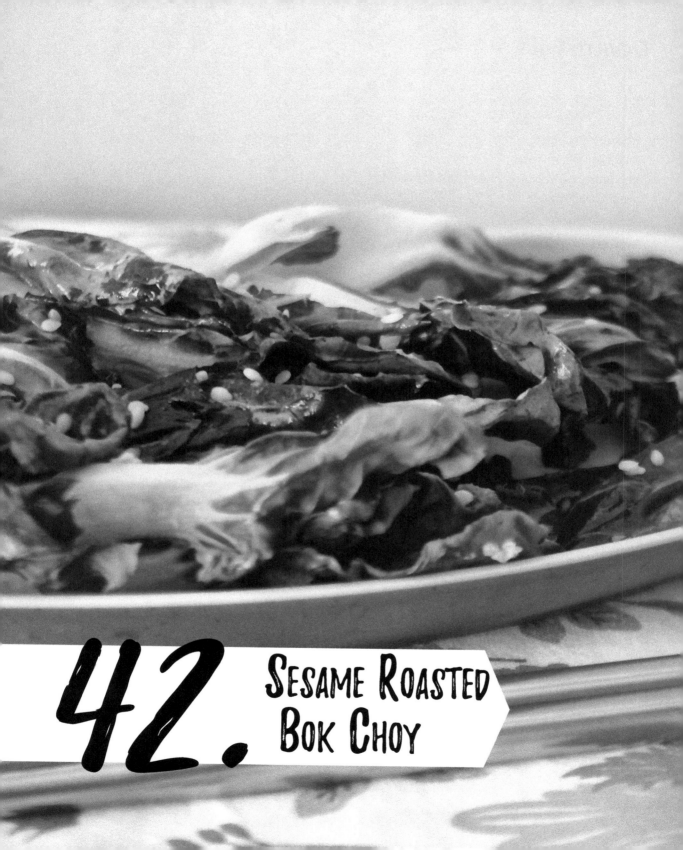

# 42. Sesame Roasted Bok Choy

# Sesame Roasted Bok Choy

SERVES 4

 WHAT YOU NEED

12 heads of baby bok choy

1 tablespoon sesame oil

2 teaspoons toasted sesame seeds

Sea salt to taste

 WHAT YOU DO

1. Preheat the oven to 400°F.

2. Thoroughly wash and trim the bok choy. On a lined baking sheet, add the bok choy and drizzle with sesame oil. Sprinkle with salt to taste.

3. Roast for about six minutes (turning each piece around at about three minutes). Top with toasted sesame seeds before serving.

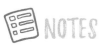 NOTES

✓ Additional topping ideas: Poppy seeds, pine nuts, drizzle of soy sauce (without high fructose corn syrup)

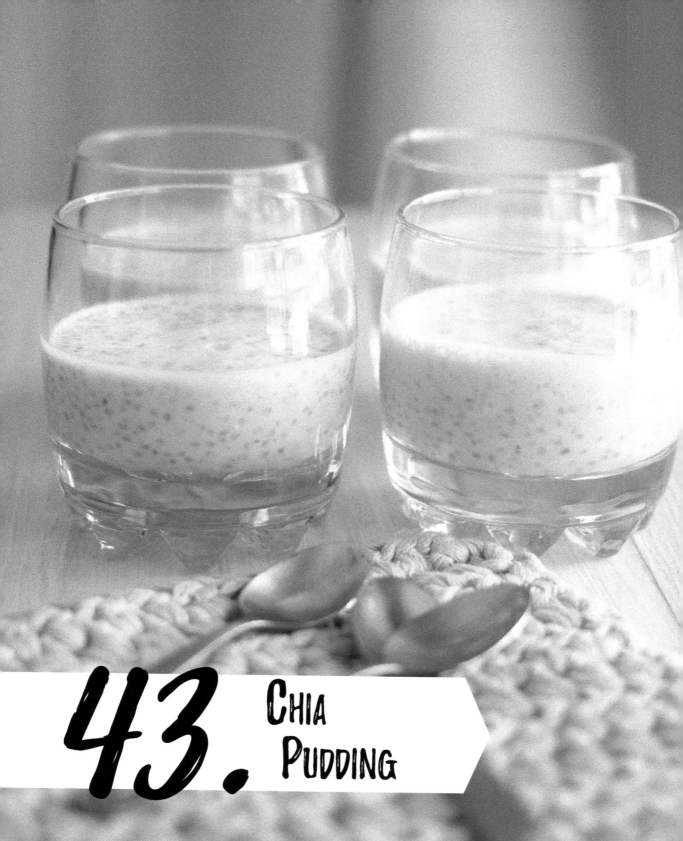

# 43. Chia Pudding

# Chia Pudding

 ## WHAT YOU NEED

½ cup chia seeds (white or black)

2 cups unsweetened macadamia milk

1-2 tablespoons pure maple syrup

### Optional Additions

1½ teaspoons cocoa powder

¼ teaspoon cinnamon

½ teaspoon vanilla extract

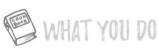 ## WHAT YOU DO

1. Combine the chia seeds, macadamia milk and maple syrup (plus any desired optional additions) in a small bowl and gently whisk with a fork.

2. Cover and refrigerate for about about five hours or until thick, stirring several times within the first hour.

3. Serve plain or with suggested toppings.

 ## NOTES

✓ Suggested toppings: strawberries, bananas, blueberries, raspberries, and shredded coconut.

✓ Don't have macadamia milk? Use rice, almond or hemp milk instead.

✓ Store refrigerated in a tightly sealed container for up to two days.

✓ If a smoother texture is preferred, blend ingredients prior to refrigerating.

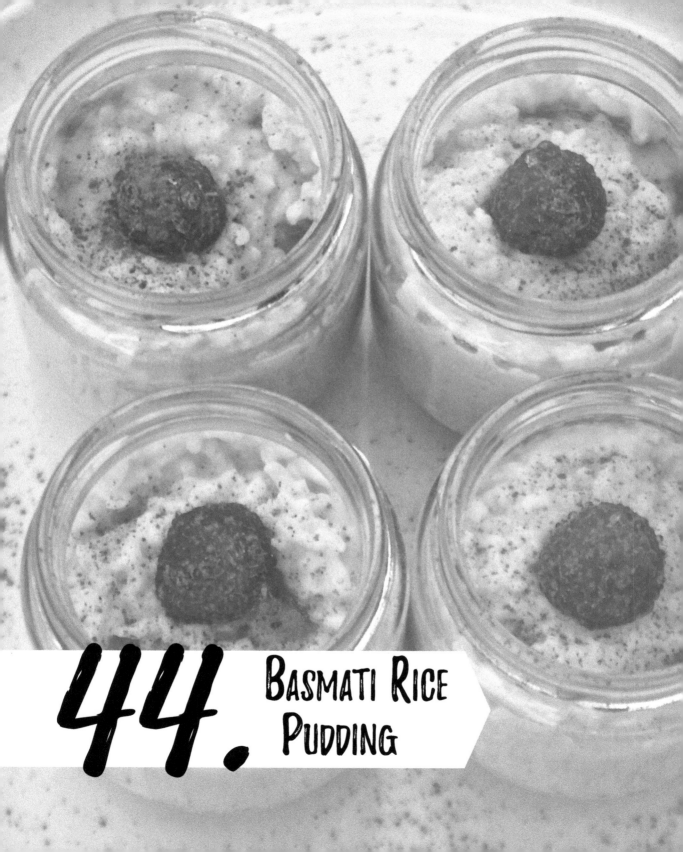

# 44.
## Basmati Rice Pudding

# BASMATI RICE PUDDING
SERVES 4-6

 WHAT YOU NEED

¾ cup basmati rice

1¾ cup full-fat coconut milk

2½ cups almond milk

1 teaspoon vanilla

½ teaspoon cinnamon

Dash nutmeg

Dash ginger

Pure maple syrup

 WHAT YOU DO

1. Combine the rice, coconut, and almond milk in a medium-sized saucepan. Bring the ingredients to a rolling boil. Once boiling, lower the heat to a simmer and cover. Cook for about 15 minutes (stirring occasionally).

2. After 15 minutes, take the cover off and continue to simmer for another 10-15 minutes (stirring occasionally) until creamy.

3. Stir in the vanilla, spices, and a little maple syrup. Cover and let rest for about five minutes prior to serving. Drizzle with maple syrup and sprinkle with cinnamon. Cover and place in the fridge (to set) for at least 3 hours prior to serving.

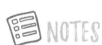 NOTES

✓ Substitute brown, white, or jasmine rice if basmati rice is not available.

✓ This style of rice pudding is more like Risgrøt, a Norwegian style of porridge my grandmother makes. Want a thicker pudding? Use less coconut and almond milk (reduce by ¼ cup).

✓ The pudding will continue to thicken the longer you cook it; it will also thicken as it rests in the fridge.

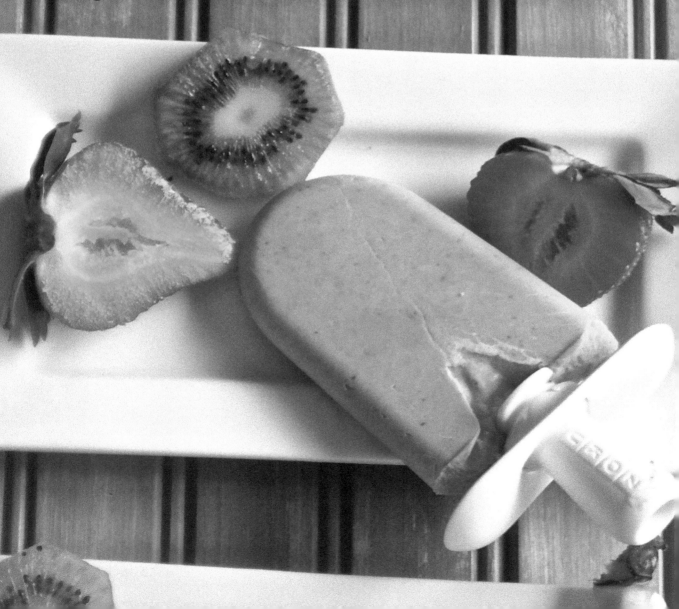

# 45. Strawberry Kiwi Banana Pops

# STRAWBERRY KIWI BANANA POPS

MAKES 4 ICE POPS

 WHAT YOU NEED

½ cup peeled and sliced kiwi

¾ cup sliced strawberries

1 banana

1¼ cup full-fat coconut milk

1-2 teaspoon brown rice syrup (optional)

 WHAT YOU DO

1. Blend all ingredients at a high speed until smooth.

2. Transfer to popsicle molds and freeze for at least six hours.

 NOTES

✓ Don't tolerate coconut milk? Try almond, hemp, or rice milk instead.

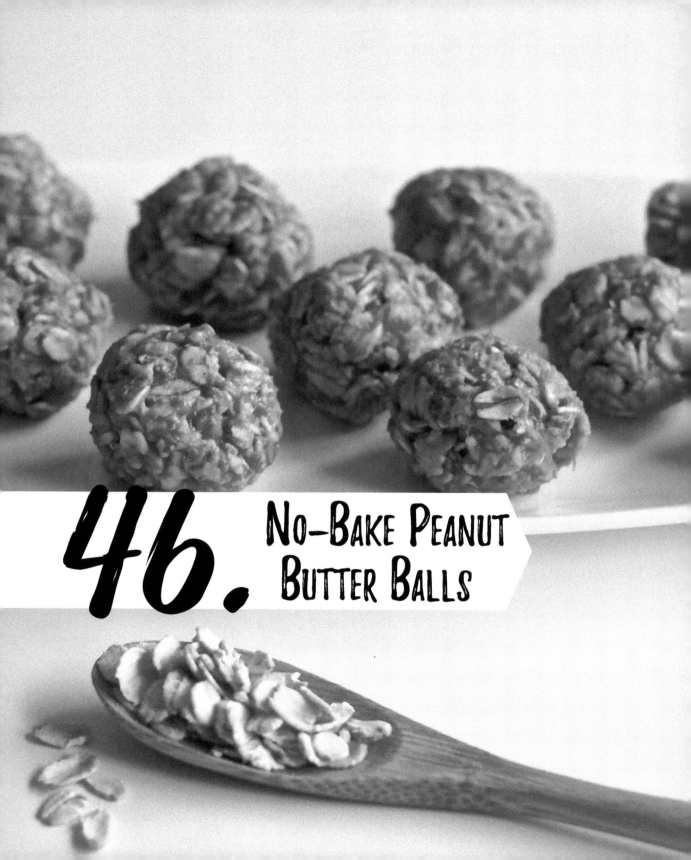

# 46.
## No-Bake Peanut Butter Balls

# No-Bake Peanut Butter Balls
MAKES 24 BALLS

 ## WHAT YOU NEED

2½ cups gluten-free rolled or quick-cooking oats

2 tablespoons pure maple syrup

¼ cup peanut butter

2 large bananas, mashed

½ teaspoon ground cinnamon

½ tablespoon vanilla

 ## WHAT YOU DO

1. In a large bowl, combine all ingredients. Place the bowl in the refrigerator (covered) for about 30 minutes.

2. Take the bowl out of the fridge and shape out 24 balls (about an inch around) and place them on a baking sheet prepped with wax paper.

3. Place the baking sheet in the refrigerator and chill for one hour. Serve or store covered in the fridge for three to five days.

 ## NOTES

✓ Not into peanut butter? Try almond butter instead.

✓ To keep this treat low FODMAP, watch portion sizes. Enjoy only one or two balls at a time.

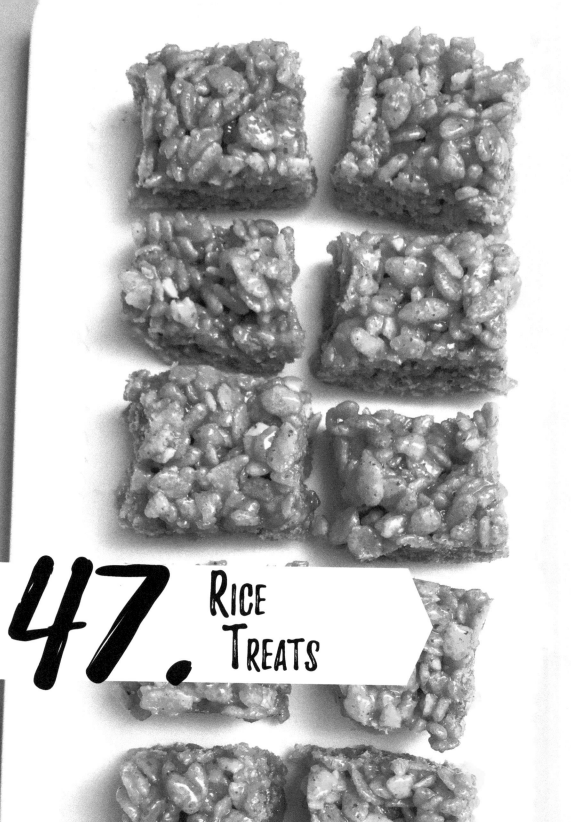

# 47. Rice Treats

# RICE TREATS

 ## WHAT YOU NEED

3 cups rice cereal
½ cup brown rice syrup
½ cup pure maple syrup

½ cup natural creamy nut butter (cashew, almond, or peanut)

 ## WHAT YOU DO

1. Start by lining an 8 x 8" high-sided baking pan with parchment paper.

2. In a medium-sized pot, combine the rice syrup, maple syrup, and nut butter over low to medium heat until smooth (about 3 minutes). Turn off the heat and add the cereal. Stir gently, mixing well until fully combined.

3. Pour the mixture onto the lined pan and use a spatula to smooth it out and press it down. Place the pan into the refrigerator for at least 40 minutes or until firm.

4. Cut the treats into 1-inch squares. Serve immediately or store in an airtight container.

 ## NOTES

✓ To keep this treat low FODMAP, watch portion sizes. Enjoy only one at a time.
✓ If you have an intolerance to gluten, read the label on your brown rice syrup and rice cereal to be sure it is gluten-free.

## READ THIS:

I've said it before, but it's important to be reminded! FODMAP research is evolving rapidly. Just as I'm ready to publish this book, new info has been released with regard to rice cereal. There seems to be some conflicting data on this particular type of cereal, but to play it safe, I'll generally advise keeping portions of crispy rice cereal below ½ cup and puffed rice cereal at ½ cup or less due to the potential presence of fructans. I decided to leave this recipe in for 2 reasons. First, these treats are easy to make and delicious. Second, over the years, I've noticed that most people react well to rice cereal. If you keep the portion size very small, they should be well-tolerated.

# 48. Cocoa Banana Smoothie

# Cocoa Banana Smoothie

SERVES 1-2

 WHAT YOU NEED

1 banana

1 teaspoon unsweetened cocoa powder

1 teaspoon pure maple syrup

2 cups unsweetened vanilla rice milk

3-5 large ice cubes (to add thickness)

 WHAT YOU DO

Place all ingredients in the blender and blend until smooth.

NOTES

✓ Don't have rice milk? Try unsweetened almond, macadamia, or hemp milk instead.

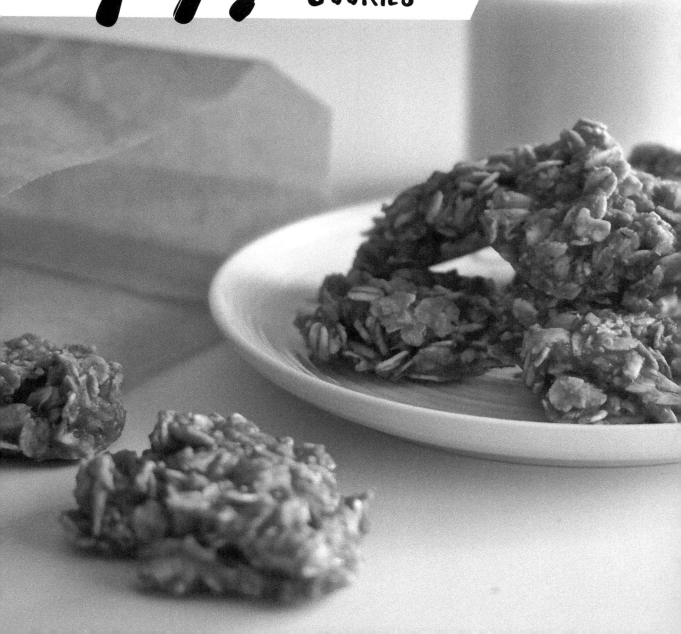

# 49.
## Oatmeal "Cookies"

# OATMEAL "COOKIES"

MAKES 12-15 COOKIES

 WHAT YOU NEED

1 cup gluten-free rolled oats

1½-2 peeled bananas

3-4 tablespoons pure maple syrup

1 teaspoon vanilla extract

¼ teaspoon cinnamon

Dash nutmeg

Dash ginger

 WHAT YOU DO

1. Preheat your oven to 350°F.

2. Placing the oats in a dry, medium-sized saucepan over medium-high heat. Stir frequently until the oats are slightly golden and fragrant (about two to three minutes). Remove from heat and let the oats cool.

3. In a separate bowl, use a masher to mash the bananas. Then, add in the toasted oats, maple syrup, vanilla, and spices. Fully combine the ingredients. Once combined, drop rounded tablespoons of the batter onto a parchment-lined cookie sheet to make about 12-15 cookies.

4. Bake in the oven for 10-12 minutes or until golden. Cool on a wire rack.

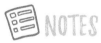 NOTES

✓ For precise measurement, a dash is equal to ⅛ teaspoon.

✓ These cookie-like treats have no butter, flour, sugar or other traditional ingredients. So, the texture and consistency is a little more chewy and the taste more natural than a typical oatmeal cookie.

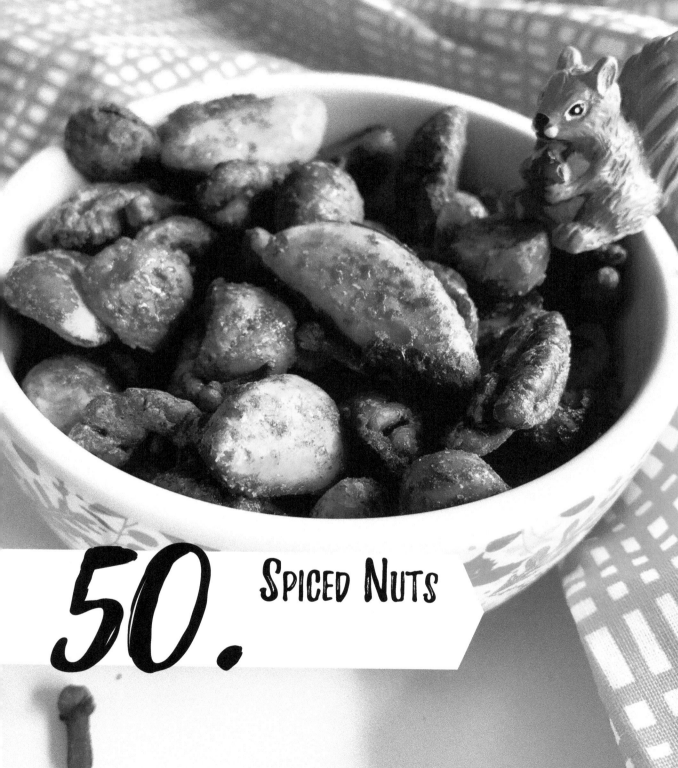

# 50. SPICED NUTS

# SPICED NUTS
MAKES 3 CUPS

 WHAT YOU NEED

3 cups mixed nuts (macadamia, brazil, pecans, walnuts, or peanuts)

1 tablespoon walnut oil

3 tablespoons pure maple syrup

1 tablespoon ground cinnamon

1 teaspoon ground ginger

1 teaspoon nutmeg

½ teaspoon ground allspice

½ teaspoon ground cloves

 WHAT YOU DO

1. Start by preheating the oven to 350°F.

2. In a small bowl, combine and mix the dry spices (cinnamon, ginger, nutmeg, allspice, and cloves).

3. In a large bowl, whisk together the walnut oil, maple syrup, and freshly mixed dry spices. Add in the nuts and stir to fully coat them.

4. Line a baking sheet with parchment paper. Add the nut mixture to the lined sheet and spread out the nuts (no clumps). Bake in the oven for about 20 minutes or until the nuts start to brown. Carefully remove the sheet from the oven and allow the nuts to cool completely. Serve cooled or store in an airtight container.

 NOTES

✓ To keep this treat low FODMAP, watch portion sizes. Enjoy only six to eight nuts at a time.

# 57. Fresh Melon Bowl

# Fresh Melon Bowl
SERVES 1

 WHAT YOU NEED

4 balls of honeydew melon (or ¼ cup diced)

8 balls of cantaloupe (or ½ cup diced)

½ teaspoon lime, zest

½ fresh lime, juice

7-8 fresh mint leaves, torn

 WHAT YOU DO

Combine ingredients.

 NOTES

✓ For extra flavor, try adding grated ginger, a pinch of sea salt, or ¼ cup diced pineapple.

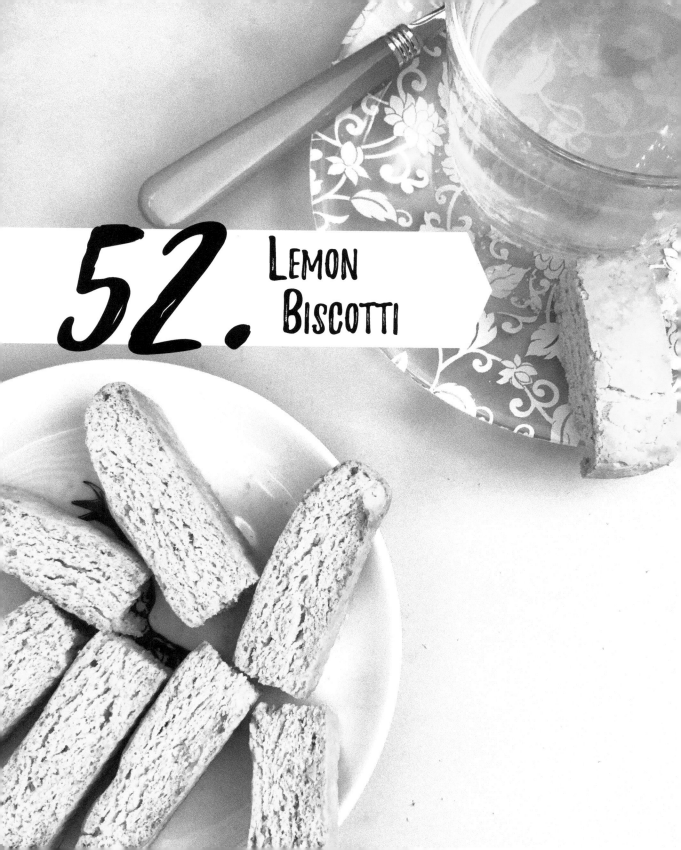

# 52. Lemon Biscotti

# LEMON BISCOTTI
MAKES 8

 WHAT YOU NEED

1¼ cup gluten-free flour*
1 teaspoon baking powder
¼ teaspoon salt
1 large lemon, zest

2 eggs, beaten
3 tablespoons pure maple syrup
2 tablespoons melted coconut oil
2 teaspoons grated ginger

 WHAT YOU DO

1. Start by preheating the oven to 325°F.

2. In a medium sized mixing bowl, combine the flour, salt, baking powder and lemon zest. In a separate mixing bowl, whisk together the beaten egg, maple syrup, coconut oil, and ginger. Add the wet ingredients to the dry. Mix well.

3. Line a baking sheet with parchment paper. Shape the mixture into a flat, rounded rectangle. Place in the oven and bake for 20-25 minutes (or until golden brown).

4. Remove from the oven and allow to cool for about 30 minutes. Once cooled, use a sharp knife to cut the biscotti into eight pieces. Be sure to use straight-down pressure and avoid a sawing motion with the knife.

5. Turn each piece on its side and bake for an additional 10 minutes. Then, flip each piece and bake again for another 10 minutes.

6. Leaving the baking sheet in, turn the oven off and allow the biscotti to fully cool and crisp for about 90 minutes. Serve or store in an airtight container.

 NOTES

✓ * If you don't use a brand of gluten-free flour that contains a binder to replace the gluten, xanthan gum is needed.
✓ Add ¾ teaspoons xanthan gum per 1 cup gluten-free flour. For this recipe, you'll need to add approximately 1½ teaspoons of xanthan gum.

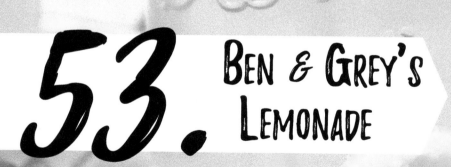

# 53.
## Ben & Grey's
## Lemonade

# BEN & GREY'S LEMONADE
## SERVES 2-4

 ## WHAT YOU NEED

2 lemons, juice

4 cups ice water

3 teaspoons of pure maple syrup

1 cup ice

 ## WHAT YOU DO

Combine ingredients by briskly stirring.

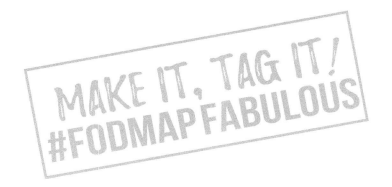

## DISCLAIMER

The FODMAP Food List and Low FODMAP Recipes have been designed according to the research available at the time this book was written. Please be mindful that FODMAP research is constantly evolving. For the latest updates, download the Monash University FODMAP Diet App.

# RECIPE NUTRIENT BREAKDOWN

## Per Serving

## BREAKFAST

### EASY BANANA FRENCH TOAST

Calories: 149
Fats: 11g
Carbs: 10.5g
Fiber: 5g
Sugar 2.5g
Protein: 8g

### COCONUT WHIPPED CREAM

Calories: 134.5
Fats: 14g
Carbs: 4g
Fiber: 0g
Sugar: 2g
Protein: 1g

### CREATE YOUR OWN FRITTATA

Calories: 107
Fats: 7g
Carbs: 0.5g
Fiber: 0g
Sugar: 0g
Protein: 9g

*Note: Breakdown depends on personalized ingredients added*

### OH-SO-GOOD OATMEAL

Calories: 109
Fats: 3g
Carbs: 18g
Fiber: 2g
Sugar: 3g
Protein: 3.5g

### MORNING GLORY SMOOTHIE

Calorie:153
Fats: 2g
Carbs: 35.5g
Fiber: 2g
Sugar: 4g
Protein: 2g

### BLUEBERRY MAPLE MUFFINS

Calories: 169
Fats: 10g
Carbs: 22g
Fiber: 2g
Sugar: 12g
Protein: 1g

## Sweet or Savory Crepes

Calories: 88
Fats: 3.5g
Carbs: 13g
Fiber: 2g
Sugar: 2g
Protein: 3g

*Note: Breakdown depends on personalized ingredients added*

## Quite a Good Quiche

Calories: 373
Fats: 21.5g
Carbs: 26g
Fiber: 3.5g
Sugar: 1.5g
Protein: 20.5g

## Blueberry Fritters

Calories: 145
Fats: 11g
Carbs: 10g
Fiber: 1g
Sugar: 4g
Protein: 4g

## Orange Pecan Granola

Calories: 361
Fats: 26g
Carbs: 29g
Fiber: 4g
Sugar: 12g
Protein: 6g

## Yogurt Parfait

*Note: Breakdown depends on personalized ingredients added*

# LUNCH/DINNER

## Stir Fried Shrimp & Rice Noodles

Calories: 453.5
Fats: 12.5g
Carbs: 52.5g
Fiber: 3g
Sugar: 0g
Protein: 30g

## Soy, Sesame Maple Salmon

Calories: 510
Fats: 25g
Carbs: 37g
Fiber: 0g
Sugar: 35.5g
Protein: 36.5g

## Kale, Orange, Feta Salad with Citrus Dressing

Calories: 74
Fats: 4g
Carbs: 8g
Fiber: 2g
Sugar: 1g
Protein: 3g

## Citrus Dressing

Calories: 35.5
Fats: 3.5g
Carbs: 1g
Fiber: 0g
Sugar: 1g
Protein: 0g

## Chicken Pecan Grape Salad Sandwich

Calories: 304
Fats: 14g
Carbs: 18g
Fiber: 11g
Sugar: 7g
Protein: 36.5g

## Rotini Pasta with Cherry Tomato & Arugula

Calories: 715
Fats: 35g
Carbs: 89.5g
Fiber: 4g
Sugar: 1.5g
Protein: 12.5g

## Chicken Fried Rice

Calories: 213
Fats: 5g
Carbs: 27g
Fiber: 1g
Sugar: 3.5g
Protein: 15g

## Chicken and Wild Rice Soup

Calories: 264
Fats: 8g
Carbs: 18g
Fiber: 3g
Sugar: 4g
Protein: 30g

## Pan-Seared Steak

Calories: 358.5
Fats: 15g
Carbs: 0.5g
Fiber: 0g
Sugar: 0g
Protein: 52g

## Turkey Tacos

Calories: 296.5
Fats: 12g
Carbs: 3.5g
Fiber: 1g
Sugar: 1.5g
Protein: 28.5g

## Veggie Noodles with Pesto & Cherry Tomatoes

Calories: 62.5
Fats: 4g
Carbs: 6g
Fiber: 1.5g
Sugar: 4g
Protein: 2g

## Pesto

Calories: 214
Fats: 22g
Carbs: 3g
Fiber: 1g
Sugar: 1g Protein: 2.5g

## Lemon Chicken

Calories: 262.5
Fats: 3.5g
Carbs: 19.5g
Fiber: 1g
Sugar: 1g
Protein: 35g

## Nicoise Salad with Tuna

Calories: 350.5

Fats: 20.5g

Carbs: 11g

Fiber: 3g

Sugar: 5g

Protein: 30g

## Roasted Red Pepper & Tomato Sauce with Pasta

Calories: 344

Fats: 5.5g

Carbs: 66.5g

Fiber: 7g

Sugar: 7g

Protein: 7g

## Stuffed Peppers

Calories: 240

Fats: 10g

Carbs: 23g

Fiber: 5g

Sugar: 3g

Protein: 15g

## Wild Rice Zucchini, Fennel, & Walnuts

Calories: 329

Fats: 22.5g

Carbs: 29g

Fiber: 6g

Sugar: 6g

Protein: 9g

## Beef & Broccoli

Calories: 242

Fats: 8g

Carbs: 13.5g

Fiber: 4g

Sugar: 4g

Protein: 29g

## Sauce

Calories: 9g

Fats: 0g

Carbs: 1g

Fiber: 0g

Sugar: 0g

Protein: 0g

## Gazpacho

Calories: 50

Fats: 0.5g

Carbs: 11g

Fiber: 2.5g

Sugar: 4.5g Protein: 2g

## Dressing

Calories: 132

Fats: 14g

Carbs: 0.5g

Fiber: 0g

Sugar: 0g

Protein: 0g

## Tomato Basil Millet

Calories: 322

Fats: 14g

Carbs: 45g

Fiber: 6g

Sugar: 0g

Protein: 7g

### Broccoli & Bacon Salad

Calories: 184
Fats: 17g
Carbs: 5.5g
Fiber: 1g
Sugar: 5g
Protein: 3.5g

### Bacon & Egg Salad

Calories: 277
Fats: 15g
Carbs: 20g
Fiber: 8.5g
Sugar: 0g
Protein: 20g

### Dressing

Calories: 164.5
Fats: 18g
Carbs: 0g
Fiber: 0g
Sugar: 0g
Protein: 0g

### Tomato Basil Millet

Calories: 322
Fats: 14g
Carbs: 45g
Fiber: 6g
Sugar: 0g
Protein: 7g

### Broccoli & Bacon Salad

Calories: 184
Fats: 17g
Carbs: 5.5g
Fiber: 1g
Sugar: 5g
Protein: 3.5g

# ON THE SIDE

### Perfect Potatoes

Calories: 111
Fats: 2g
Carbs: 19g
Fiber: 1.5g
Sugar: 0g
Protein: 2.5g

### Pineapple Rice

Calories: 122
Fats: 1.5g
Carbs: 25g
Fiber: 1g
Sugar: 3g
Protein: 3g

## Lemon & Parsley Fingerling Potatoes

Calorie: 156
Fats: 7.5g
Carbs: 21g
Fiber: 2.5g
Sugar: 1g
Protein: 2.5g

## Easy Wok Vegetable (with Peanuts)

Calories: 154
Fats: 8.5g
Carbs: 14g
Fiber: 2g
Sugar: 2.5g
Protein: 5.5g

## Without Peanuts

Calories: 82.5
Fats: 2.5g
Carbs: 11g
Fiber: 1g
Sugar: 2g
Protein: 2.5g

## Cilantro Lime Brown Rice

Calories: 148.5
Fats: 4g
Carbs: 25g
Fiber: 2g
Sugar: 0g
Protein: 2.5g

## Pineapple & Cucumber Salad

Calories: 162
Fats: 4g
Carbs: 34g
Fiber: 4g
Sugar: 24g
Protein: 2g

## Spiced Popcorn

Calories: 199
Fats: 12g
Carbs: 21g
Fiber: 3.5g
Sugar: 0g
Protein: 3g

## Kiwi Fennel Salad

Calories: 181
Fats: 6.5g
Carbs: 32g
Fiber: 8g
Sugar: 19g
Protein: 5g

## Orange & Mint Dressing

Calories: 395
Fats: 41g
Carbs: 9g
Fiber: 2g
Sugar: 6g
Protein: 1g

## Homemade Potato Chips

Calories: 176
Fats: 9.5g
Carbs: 22g
Fiber: 1.5g
Sugar: 2g
Protein: 2g

## Tomato Salad

Calories: 133
Fats: 12g
Carbs: 2g
Fiber: 1g
Sugar: 2g
Protein: .5g

## Deviled Eggs

Calories: 84
Fats: 1.5g
Carbs: 0g
Fiber: 0g
Sugar: 0g
Protein: 1.5g

## Sesame Roasted Bok Choy

Calories: 120
Fats: 3.5g
Carbs: 9g
Fiber: 0g
Sugar: 0g
Protein: 3g

# TREATS

## Chia Pudding

Calories: 222
Fats: 20g
Carbs: 34g
Fiber: 12g
Sugar: 9g
Protein: 5g

## No Bake Peanut Butter Balls

Calories: 71
Fats: 2g
Carbs: 11g
Fiber: 1.5g
Sugar: 3g
Protein: 2g

## Basmati Rice Pudding

Calories: 258
Fats: 23g
Carbs: 12g
Fiber: 1g
Sugar: 0g
Protein: 4g

## Rice Treats

Calories: 143
Fats: 4g
Carbs: 25.5g
Fiber: 0g
Sugar: 16g
Protein: 2.5g

## Strawberry Kiwi Banana Pops

Calories: 188.5
Fats: 15.5g
Carbs: 14g
Fiber: 2g
Sugar: 7.5g
Protein: 2g

## Cocoa Banana Smoothie

Calories: 76
Fats: 1.5g
Carbs: 16.5g
Fiber: 2g
Sugar: 9.5g
Protein: 1g

## Oatmeal Cookies

Calories: 54
Fats: 0.5g
Carbs: 12g
Fiber: 1g
Sugar: 2g
Protein: 1g

## Spiced Nuts

Calories: 933
Fats: 76g
Carbs: 54g
Fiber: 15g
Sugar: 13g
Protein: 24g

## Fresh Melon Bowl

Calories: 68
Fats: 0g
Carbs: 17g
Fiber: 2g
Sugar: 15g
Protein: 1g

## Lemon Biscotti

Calories: 166
Fats: 7g
Carbs: 26g
Fiber: 3g
Sugar: 7.5g
Protein: 4g

## Ben & Grey's Lemonade

Calories: 18
Fats: 0g
Carbs: 5g
Fiber: 0g
Sugar: 4g
Protein: 0g

# REFERENCES

Monash University Diet App. (2018) Monash University (Version 2.0.10) [Mobile Application Software] Retrieved from http://itunes.apple.com

Dolan R, Chey WD, Eswaran S. The role of diet in the management of irritable bowel syndrome: a focus on FODMAPs. Expert Rev Gastroenterol Hepatol. 2018 May 18:1-9.

Eswaran S, Farida JP, Green J, Miller JD, Chey WD. Nutrition in the management of gastrointestinal diseases and disorders: the evidence for the low FODMAP diet. Curr Opin Pharmacol. 2017 Dec;37:151-157.

Testa A, Imperatore N, Rispo A, Rea M, Tortora R, Nardone OM, et al. Beyond Irritable Bowel Syndrome: The Efficacy of the Low Fodmap Diet for Improving Symptoms in Inflammatory Bowel Diseases and Celiac Disease. Dig Dis. 2018 May 15:1-10.

Mazzawi T, El-Salhy M. Effect of diet and individual dietary guidance on gastrointestinal endocrine cells in patients with irritable bowel syndrome (Review).Int J Mol Med. 2017 Oct;40(4):943-952.

Dieterich W, Schuppan D, Schink M, Schwappacher R, Wirtz S, Agaimy A, et al. Influence of low FODMAP and gluten-free diets on disease activity and intestinal microbiota in patients with non-celiac gluten sensitivity. Clin Nutr. 2018 Apr 4. pii: S0261-5614(18)30129-8.

Valeur J, Småstuen MC, Knudsen T, Lied GA, Røseth AG. Exploring Gut Microbiota Composition as an Indicator of Clinical Response to Dietary FODMAP Restriction in Patients with Irritable Bowel Syndrome. Dig Dis Sci. 2018 Feb;63(2):429-436.

Snipe RMJ, Khoo A, Kitic CM, Gibson PR, Costa RJS. The low FODMAP diet in the management of irritable bowel syndrome: an evidence-based review of FODMAP restriction, reintroduction and personalisation in clinical practice. J Hum Nutr Diet. 2018 Apr;31(2):239-255.

Zhou SY, Gillilland M 3rd, Wu X, Leelasinjaroen P, Zhang G, Zhou H. FODMAP diet modulates visceral nociception by lipopolysaccharide-mediated intestinal inflammation and barrier dysfunction. J Clin Invest. 2018 Jan 2;128(1):267-280.

Barbalho SM,Goulart RA, Aranão ALC, de Oliveira PGC. Inflammatory Bowel Diseases and Fermentable Oligosaccharides, Disaccharides, Monosaccharides, and Polyols: An Overview. J Med Food. 2018 Jan 12. doi: 10.1089/jmf.2017.0120.

Diduch BK. Gastrointestinal Conditions in the Female Athlete. Clin Sports Med. 2017 Oct;36(4):655-669.

Elisabet Johannesson, Gisela Ringström, Hasse Abrahamsson, and Riadh Sadik. Intervention to increase physical activity in irritable bowel syndrome shows long-term positive effects. World J Gastroenterol. 2015 Jan 14; 21(2): 600–608.

Amy E. Foxx-Orenstein. New and emerging therapies for the treatment of irritable bowel syndrome: an update for gastroenterologists. Therap Adv Gastroenterol. 2016 May; 9(3): 354–375.

Full-Young Chang. Irritable bowel syndrome: The evolution of multi-dimensional looking and multidisciplinary treatments. World J Gastroenterol. 2014 Mar 14; 20(10): 2499–2514.

Soo-Kyung Lim, Seung Jin Yoo, Dae Lim Koo, Chae A Park, Han Jun Ryu, Yong Jin Jung, et al. Stress and sleep quality in doctors working on-call shifts are associated with functional gastrointestinal disorders. World J Gastroenterol. 2017 May 14; 23(18): 3330–3337.

# INDEX

# Z

CPSIA information can be obtained
at www.ICGtesting.com
Printed in the USA
BVHW021400291118
534352BV00013B/113/P

9 781732 450202